Pharmacy Technician Certification Exam
PRACTICE QUESTION
WORKBOOK

1,000 Comprehensive
Practice Questions

Renee Bonsell, PharmD, RPh

ISBN: 0999510533
ISBN-13: 978-0999510537

CONTENTS

DOMAIN 1

PHARMACOLOGY

QUESTIONS

1. A thyroid-stimulating hormone (TSH) test should be performed periodically if a patient is taking which of the following medications?

    a. Levothyroxine
    b. Montelukast
    c. Propranolol
    d. Furosemide

2. Which of the following medications is a rapid-acting insulin?

    a. Insulin glargine (Lantus)
    b. Insulin lispro (Humalog)
    c. Insulin detemir (Levemir)
    d. Regular insulin (Humulin)

3. Which of the following medications is an example of a beta-blocker?

    a. Lisinopril
    b. Sertraline
    c. Carvedilol
    d. Hydrochlorothiazide

4. Protease inhibitors, integrase inhibitors, and nucleoside reverse transcriptase inhibitors can be used in the treatment of _____.

    a. HIV/AIDS
    b. influenza
    c. herpes
    d. hepatitis

5. Zoloft is the brand name for which of the following medications?

    a. Sucralfate
    b. Diltiazem
    c. Sertraline
    d. Benazepril

6. Warfarin levels can be affected by which of the following foods?

    a. Dairy products
    b. Soda
    c. Leafy greens
    d. Water

7. A drug with the suffix "-pril" belongs to which class of medications?

    a. ARBs
    b. Beta-blockers
    c. Diuretics
    d. ACE inhibitors

8. Zolpidem is indicated for the treatment of which of the following conditions?

    a. Depression
    b. Anxiety
    c. Pain
    d. Insomnia

9. Tamiflu, Relenza, and Rapivab belong to which pharmacologic category?

    a. Antidiarrheal
    b. Antiviral
    c. Antibiotic
    d. Antiprotozoal

10. A therapeutically equivalent medication must have the same strength, dosage form, route of administration, and _____.

    a. active ingredients
    b. inactive ingredients
    c. active and inactive ingredients
    d. color and size

11. Which of the following side effects commonly occurs with the use of phenazopyridine?

    a. Insomnia
    b. Fluid retention
    c. Constipation
    d. Discoloration of the urine

12. Which of the following medications is an H2 receptor antagonist?

    a. Omeprazole
    b. Lansoprazole
    c. Cimetidine
    d. Sucralfate

13. Latanoprost is used for the treatment of which ocular condition?

    a. Conjunctivitis
    b. Corneal abrasion
    c. Macular degeneration
    d. Glaucoma

14. Members of the triptan medication class are used for the treatment of _____.

    a. migraine headaches
    b. epilepsy
    c. hypertension
    d. GERD

15. Glyburide is a member of which hypoglycemic medication class?

    a. Biguanide
    b. Alpha-glucosidase inhibitor
    c. Thiazolidinedione
    d. Sulfonylurea

16. Women who are pregnant should avoid the use of which of the following medications?

    a. Clindamycin
    b. Amoxicillin
    c. Tetracycline
    d. Penicillin

17. Fluoxetine is the generic name for which of the following SSRIs?

    a. Paxil
    b. Celexa
    c. Lexapro
    d. Prozac

18. All but which of the following medications is classified as an NSAID?

    a. Naproxen
    b. Ibuprofen
    c. Aspirin
    d. Acetaminophen

19. **Antibiotics can reduce the effectiveness of which of the following classes of medications?**

    a. Analgesics
    b. Statins
    c. Oral contraceptives
    d. Antifungals

20. **Enoxaparin is the generic name for which of the following medications?**

    a. Lovenox
    b. Heparin
    c. Arixtra
    d. Xarelto

21. **All but which of the following is an example of an antiarrhythmic medication?**

    a. Amiodarone
    b. Quinapril
    c. Propafenone
    d. Flecainide

22. **Dairy products can affect the absorption of which of the following antibiotics?**

    a. Cephalexin
    b. Penicillin
    c. Trimethoprim
    d. Tetracycline

23. **Losartan is the generic name for which of the following ARBs?**

    a. Cozaar
    b. Avapro
    c. Micardis
    d. Benicar

24. **All but which of the following medications is used for the treatment of angina?**

    a. Nitroglycerin
    b. Montelukast
    c. Isosorbide mononitrate
    d. Isosorbide dinitrate

25. Which of the following medications is the generic name for Lotrel?

a. Amlodipine-benazepril
b. Amlodipine-atorvastatin
c. Losartan-hydrochlorothiazide
d. Lisinopril-hydrochlorothiazide

26. A patient taking a monoamine oxidase inhibitor (MAOI) should avoid foods and beverages that contain _____.

a. calcium
b. vitamin K
c. tyramine
d. iron

27. Which of the following vitamins is water soluble?

a. Vitamin A
b. Vitamin C
c. Vitamin D
d. Vitamin E

28. Which of the following medications should be avoided or used with caution in patients who have a sulfa allergy?

a. Hydrochlorothiazide
b. Carvedilol
c. Quinapril
d. All of the above

29. All but which of the following medications is used topically for the treatment of acne vulgaris?

a. Adapalene
b. Salicylic acid
c. Isotretinoin
d. Benzoyl peroxide

30. Olanzapine is the generic name for which of the following medications?

a. Risperdal
b. Geodon
c. Abilify
d. Zyprexa

31. Depression can be treated with which of the following classes of medications?

    a. Statins
    b. COX-2 inhibitors
    c. SSRIs
    d. Beta-blockers

32. All but which of the following ADHD medications is classified as a stimulant?

    a. Strattera
    b. Vyvanse
    c. Adderall
    d. Ritalin

33. Tadalafil is the generic name for which erectile dysfunction drug?

    a. Cialis
    b. Levitra
    c. Viagra
    d. Stendra

34. Amlodipine is a member of which drug classification?

    a. ARB
    b. Diuretic
    c. Calcium channel blocker
    d. Beta-blocker

35. Which of the following medications should be taken on an empty stomach?

    a. Prednisone
    b. Methylprednisolone
    c. Levothyroxine
    d. Metformin

36. Diovan HCT is a combination of which of the following medications?

    a. Valsartan and hydrochlorothiazide
    b. Olmesartan and hydrochlorothiazide
    c. Valsartan and hydralazine
    d. Irbesartan and hydrochlorothiazide

37. Which of the following medications is used for the treatment of hypothyroidism?

a. Methimazole
b. Propylthiouracil
c. Liothyronine
d. Primidone

38. Which of the following medications is classified as an antiviral?

a. Fluconazole
b. Moxifloxacin
c. Acyclovir
d. Nystatin

39. All but which of the following medications is classified as an antihistamine?

a. Loratadine
b. Montelukast
c. Chlorpheniramine
d. Cetirizine

40. Which of the following medications is a potassium supplement?

a. Caltrate
b. Folbee
c. VP-Zel
d. Klor-Con

41. Ibuprofen is the active ingredient in _____.

a. Advil
b. Aleve
c. Tylenol
d. Bufferin

42. Which of the following medications is classified as a bronchodilator?

a. Zafirlukast
b. Albuterol
c. Loratadine
d. Budesonide

43. Amiodarone is indicated for the treatment of which of the following conditions?

a. Angina
b. Arrhythmia
c. Hypertension
d. Ulcerative colitis

44. Memantine is the generic name for which of the following medications?

a. Namenda
b. Aricept
c. Razadyne
d. Exelon

45. Which of the following is defined as the study of what a drug does to the body?

a. Pharmacodynamics
b. Pharmacology
c. Pharmacokinetics
d. Pharmaceutics

46. Proton pump inhibitors are used to decrease the production of which of the following substances in the body?

a. Thyroid hormone
b. Uric acid
c. Leukotrienes
d. Stomach acid

47. Tamoxifen is a hormone agent used for the prevention and treatment of which of the following types of cancer?

a. Prostate
b. Lung
c. Breast
d. Pancreatic

48. Which of the following antibiotics can cause photosensitivity?

a. Ciprofloxacin
b. Sulfamethoxazole
c. Doxycycline
d. All of the above

49. Patients taking anticoagulants should use which of the following medications with caution?

a. Montelukast
b. Loratadine
c. Aspirin
d. Metformin

50. Patients taking a statin should avoid which of the following foods?

a. Milk
b. Grapefruit
c. Bananas
d. Leafy greens

ANSWER KEY

1. A
A thyroid-stimulating hormone (TSH) test should be performed periodically if a patient is taking levothyroxine.

2. B
Insulin lispro (Humalog) is a rapid-acting insulin.

3. C
Carvedilol is an example of a beta-blocker.

4. A
Protease inhibitors, integrase inhibitors, and nucleoside reverse transcriptase inhibitors can be used in the treatment of HIV/AIDS.

5. C
Zoloft is the brand name for sertraline.

6. C
Warfarin levels can be affected by leafy greens.

7. D
A drug with the suffix "-pril" belongs to the ACE inhibitor class.

8. D
Zolpidem is indicated for the treatment of insomnia.

9. B
Tamiflu, Relenza, and Rapivab are antiviral medications.

10. A
A therapeutically equivalent medication must have the same strength, dosage form, route of administration, and active ingredients.

11. D
A common side effect of phenazopyridine is discoloration of the urine.

12. C
Cimetidine is an H2 receptor antagonist.

13. D
Latanoprost is used for the treatment of glaucoma.

14. A
Members of the triptan medication class are used for the treatment of migraine headaches.

15. D
Glyburide is a member of the sulfonylurea hypoglycemic medication class.

16. C
Women who are pregnant should avoid the use of tetracycline.

17. D
Fluoxetine is the generic name for Prozac.

18. D
Naproxen, ibuprofen, and aspirin are classified as NSAIDs.

19. C
Antibiotics can reduce the effectiveness of oral contraceptives.

20. A
Enoxaparin is the generic name for Lovenox.

21. B
Amiodarone, propafenone, and flecainide are examples of antiarrhythmic medications.

22. D
Dairy products can affect the absorption of tetracycline.

23. A
Losartan is the generic name for Cozaar.

24. B
Nitroglycerin, isosorbide mononitrate, and isosorbide dinitrate are used for the treatment of angina.

25. A
Amlodipine-benazepril is the generic name for Lotrel.

26. C
A patient taking a monoamine oxidase inhibitor (MAOI) should avoid foods and beverages that contain tyramine.

27. B
Vitamin C is water soluble.

28. A
Hydrochlorothiazide should be avoided or used with caution in patients who have a sulfa allergy.

29. C
Adapalene, salicylic acid, and benzoyl peroxide are used topically for the treatment of acne vulgaris.

30. D
Olanzapine is the generic name for Zyprexa.

31. C
Depression can be treated with SSRIs.

32. A
Vyvanse, Adderall, and Ritalin are ADHD medications that are classified as stimulants.

33. A
Tadalafil is the generic name for Cialis.

34. C
Amlodipine is a calcium channel blocker.

35. C
Levothyroxine should be taken on an empty stomach.

36. A
Diovan HCT is a combination of valsartan and hydrochlorothiazide.

37. C
Liothyronine is used for the treatment of hypothyroidism.

38. C
Acyclovir is classified as an antiviral.

39. B
Loratadine, chlorpheniramine, and cetirizine are classified as antihistamines.

40. D
Klor-Con is a potassium supplement.

41. A
Ibuprofen is the active ingredient in Advil.

42. B
Albuterol is classified as a bronchodilator.

43. B
Amiodarone is indicated for the treatment of arrhythmias.

44. A
Memantine is the generic name for Namenda.

45. A
Pharmacodynamics is the study of what a drug does to the body.

46. D
Proton pump inhibitors are used to decrease the production of stomach acid.

47. C
Tamoxifen is a hormone agent used for the prevention and treatment of breast cancer.

48. D
Ciprofloxacin, sulfamethoxazole, and doxycycline are antibiotics that can cause photo-sensitivity.

49. C
Patients taking anticoagulants should use aspirin with caution.

50. B
Patients taking a statin should avoid grapefruit.

DOMAIN 2

PHARMACY LAW AND REGULATIONS

QUESTIONS

1. The law requiring pharmacists to perform a prospective drug review, provide patient counseling, and maintain patient records is the _____.

   a. Resource Conservation and Recovery Act
   b. Medicare Prescription Drug, Improvement, and Modernization Act of 2003
   c. Health Insurance Portability and Accountability Act of 1996
   d. Omnibus Budget Reconciliation Act of 1990

2. Pharmacy employees who handle a hazardous chemical should refer to which of the following resources to find information about the hazards of the product and advised safety precautions?

   a. Safety Data Sheet (SDS)
   b. United States Pharmacopeia
   c. Orange Book
   d. The Merck Manual

3. Prescriptions for non-controlled medications are valid for _____ from the date written.

   a. three months
   b. six months
   c. nine months
   d. twelve months

4. Which of the following is true regarding mailing controlled substances via the United States Postal Service?

   a. Schedule II controlled substances cannot be mailed.
   b. Schedule III-V controlled substances cannot be mailed.
   c. Only Schedule V controlled substances are permitted to be mailed.
   d. All controlled substances are permitted to be mailed.

5. The third segment of an NDC number identifies which of the following?

   a. Drug manufacturer (labeler)
   b. Package size and type (package code)
   c. Strength, dosage form, and formulation (product code)
   d. Expiration date

6. All but which of the following are examples of a Schedule V controlled substance?

a. Tylenol with codeine
b. Robitussin AC
c. Phenergan with codeine
d. Lomotil

7. A prescription for a Schedule II controlled substance may be faxed to a pharmacy in all but which of the following scenarios?

a. The patient is in hospice care.
b. The patient is a resident of a long-term care facility.
c. The prescription is for a Schedule II controlled substance to be compounded for direct patient administration via parenteral, intravenous, intramuscular, subcutaneous, or intraspinal infusion.
d. The patient is being discharged from a hospital.

8. How often must a pharmacy complete an inventory of controlled substances according to federal law?

a. Every year
b. Every two years
c. Every three years
d. Every four years

9. Which chapter of the *United States Pharmacopeia* provides guidance for the compounding of non-sterile formulations for human or animal administration?

a. USP <795>
b. USP <797>
c. USP <1160>
d. USP <1176>

10. A drug recall in which the use or exposure of the violative substance is not likely to cause adverse health consequences would be in which of the following recall classes?

a. Class I recall
b. Class II recall
c. Class III recall
d. None of the above

11. Which of the following organizations develops standards regarding the identity, strength, quality, and purity of medications and dietary supplements?

a. FDA
b. TJC
c. USP
d. DEA

12. An oral order for a Schedule II controlled substance is permitted _____.

a. if the patient is a resident of a long-term care facility
b. in an emergency situation
c. if the patient is terminally ill
d. if a prescription is being refilled

13. Which organization evaluates and accredits health care organizations and programs in the United States?

a. FDA
b. OSHA
c. TJC
d. CMS

14. Medications that have no currently accepted medical use and a high potential for abuse are in which of the following drug schedules?

a. Schedule I
b. Schedule II
c. Schedule III
d. Schedule V

15. Which of the following laws requires that new drugs must be proven safe and have FDA approval granted prior to marketing?

a. Food, Drug, and Cosmetic Act of 1938
b. Pure Food and Drug Act of 1906
c. Durham-Humphrey Amendment of 1951
d. Controlled Substances Act

16. Which of the following should be the last digit of Dr. Brent Cole's DEA number if it begins with BC372514_?

a. 2
b. 5
c. 8
d. 9

17. **In which of the following scenarios is partially filling a Schedule II controlled substance permitted?**

    a. Schedule II controlled substances can never be partially filled.
    b. The pharmacy is out of stock of the particular medication.
    c. There are no restrictions on partially filling Schedule II controlled substances.
    d. None of the above

18. **The second segment of an NDC number identifies which of the following?**

    a. Package size and type (package code)
    b. Drug manufacturer (labeler)
    c. Strength, dosage form, and formulation (product code)
    d. Expiration date

19. **According to federal law, a prescription for a Schedule II controlled substance must be filled within how many days or months of the date written?**

    a. Seven days
    b. Thirty days
    c. Ninety days
    d. Six months

20. **Which of the following reference books is required to be in every pharmacy?**

    a. United States Pharmacopeia
    b. American Drug Index
    c. Facts and Comparisons
    d. Orange Book

21. **Chemotherapeutic agents should be prepared in which of the following types of environment?**

    a. Compounding Aseptic Isolator
    b. Recirculating Compounding Aseptic Isolator
    c. Class II Biological Safety Cabinet (Vertical Laminar Flow Hood)
    d. Buffer area

22. **Which of the following laws separated drugs into prescription and over-the-counter categories?**

    a. Durham-Humphrey Amendment of 1951
    b. Kefauver-Harris Amendment of 1962
    c. Food, Drug, and Cosmetic Act of 1938
    d. Pure Food and Drug Act of 1906

23. Which of the following medications are exempt from the requirements of the Poison Prevention Packaging Act of 1970?

a. Penicillin
b. Sublingual nitroglycerin tablets
c. Prednisolone
d. Methotrexate

24. The first segment of an NDC number identifies which of the following?

a. Package size and type (package code)
b. Expiration date
c. Strength, dosage form, and formulation (product code)
d. Drug manufacturer (labeler)

25. If a patient requests that medication be dispensed in a "non-child-resistant" container, the pharmacy should do which of the following?

a. Document the information in the patient's record
b. Receive authorization from the prescriber
c. Refuse to dispense the medication
d. No further action is necessary

26. Which of the following laws classified controlled substances into one of five categories based on their abuse potential and accepted medical use?

a. Narcotic Drug Act of 1914
b. Orphan Drug Act of 1983
c. Food, Drug, and Cosmetic Act of 1938
d. Comprehensive Drug Abuse Prevention and Control Act of 1970

27. Which of the following laws established the provision that all patient medical records and other personal health information must be kept private?

a. Medicare Prescription Drug, Improvement, and Modernization Act of 2003
b. Health Insurance Portability and Accountability Act of 1996
c. Omnibus Budget and Reconciliation Act of 1990
d. Kefauver-Harris Amendment of 1962

28. The Combat Methamphetamine Epidemic Act of 2005 regulates the sale of over-the-counter products containing all but which of the following?

a. Phentermine
b. Pseudoephedrine
c. Ephedrine
d. Phenylpropanolamine

29. **Which of the following regulations are included in the Occupational Safety and Health Act of 1970?**

    a. Sets standards to ensure that employers are providing safe and healthy work-places
    b. Requires that chemical manufacturers provide to the purchaser Safety Data Sheets for hazardous chemicals
    c. Gives employees the right to file a complaint with OSHA regarding safety and health conditions in their workplace
    d. All of the above

30. **iPledge is a Risk Evaluation and Mitigation Strategy (REMS) program that pertains to which of the following medications?**

    a. Thalidomide
    b. Isotretinoin
    c. Clozapine
    d. Lithium

31. **Which of the following laws prohibits the re-importation of drugs into the United States and regulates the sale of samples?**

    a. Hatch-Waxman Act of 1984
    b. Prescription Drug Marketing Act of 1987
    c. Resource Conservation and Recovery Act
    d. Pure Food and Drug Act of 1906

32. **Prescriptions for drugs in Schedules III-V may be transferred between pharmacies how many times according to federal law?**

    a. One time
    b. Two times
    c. Three times
    d. Unlimited times

33. **Which of the following regulatory agencies establishes guidelines for the disposal of hazardous waste?**

    a. DEA
    b. FDA
    c. EPA
    d. OSHA

34. A forged prescription may display which of the following characteristics?

a. Prescription is written in different color inks
b. Prescription appears to be photocopied
c. The drug prescribed differs in quantity, directions, or dosage from typical medical usage
d. All of the above

35. According to USP <797>, pharmacy personnel who compound low- and medium-risk level sterile products must have their aseptic technique evaluated how often?

a. Monthly
b. Quarterly
c. Semi-annually
d. Annually

36. A drug label that does not contain adequate directions for use would be in violation of which of the following federal laws?

a. Poison Prevention Packaging Act of 1970
b. Drug Listing Act of 1972
c. Prescription Drug Marketing Act of 1987
d. Food, Drug, and Cosmetic Act of 1938

37. The Combat Methamphetamine Epidemic Act of 2005 requires that the logbook of pseudoephedrine sales includes all but which of the following information?

a. Product name and quantity
b. Purchaser name and address
c. Method of payment
d. Date and time of sale

38. Prescribers must have a DEA number in order to write prescriptions for _____.

a. intravenous medications
b. controlled substances
c. pseudoephedrine-containing medications
d. all prescription medications

39. All but which of the following are required for the over-the-counter sale of select Schedule V medications?

a. The purchaser must be at least 21 years of age.
b. The purchaser must complete the Exempt Narcotic Book.
c. No more than one container can be sold to the same purchaser within a 48-hour period.
d. The product must be sold in the original manufacturer's container.

40. No more than _____ refills are permitted for a Schedule III-V controlled substance prescription.

a. two
b. three
c. four
d. five

41. Which of the following DEA forms is used to order Schedule II medications?

a. Form 41
b. Form 106
c. Form 222
d. Form 224

42. According to federal law, prescriptions for non-controlled medications must initially be filled within _____ of the date written.

a. thirty days
b. ninety days
c. six months
d. twelve months

43. Which of the following is an example of a Schedule II controlled substance?

a. Acetaminophen-hydrocodone
b. Acetaminophen-codeine
c. Diazepam
d. Phenobarbital

44. All but which of the following is true regarding the issuance of multiple prescriptions for a particular Schedule II controlled substance from a prescriber to a patient?

a. Each prescription must be issued on a separate prescription blank.
b. The prescriber must indicate the earliest date each prescription can be filled.
c. The patient may receive up to a twelve month supply.
d. The issuance of multiple prescriptions must be permitted by applicable state laws.

45. Generally, a generic substitution can be made for a drug if the generic product meets which of the following criteria?

a. Same inactive ingredient(s)
b. Same dose but different dosage form
c. Same route of administration
d. All of the above

46. Which of the following chapters of the *United States Pharmacopeia* provides guidance for the compounding of sterile products?

a. USP <795>
b. USP <797>
c. USP <1163>
d. USP <1176>

47. Pharmacy records such as prescriptions, controlled substance inventory records, and invoices must be able to be retrieved within how long of a request?

a. 24 hours
b. 36 hours
c. 48 hours
d. 72 hours

48. Which of the following federal agencies administers the Medicare and Medicaid programs?

a. CMS
b. FDA
c. DEA
d. OSHA

49. A prescriber who is authorized to prescribe Subutex or Suboxone for the treatment of opioid addiction must have a special DEA number that starts with which of the following letters?

a. M
b. F
c. X
d. P

50. Information on the generic equivalence of drugs can be found in which of the following resources?

a. The Merck Manual
b. Remington: The Science and Practice of Pharmacy
c. Physicians' Desk Reference
d. Orange Book

ANSWER KEY

1. D
The Omnibus Budget Reconciliation Act of 1990 requires pharmacists to perform a prospective drug review, provide patient counseling, and maintain patient records.

2. A
Pharmacy employees who handle a hazardous chemical should refer to the product's Safety Data Sheet (SDS) to find information about the hazards of the product and advised safety precautions.

3. D
Prescriptions for non-controlled medications are valid for twelve months from the date written.

4. D
The United States Postal Service permits the mailing of any controlled substance.

5. B
The third segment of an NDC number identifies the package size and type (package code).

6. A
Robitussin AC, Phenergan with codeine, and Lomotil are examples of Schedule V controlled substances.

7. D
A prescription for a Schedule II controlled substance may be faxed to a pharmacy if the patient is in hospice care, the patient is a resident of a long term-care facility, or the prescription is for a Schedule II controlled substance to be compounded for direct patient administration via parenteral, intravenous, intramuscular, subcutaneous, or intraspinal infusion.

8. B
A pharmacy must complete an inventory of controlled substances every two years according to federal law.

9. A
USP <795> provides guidance for the compounding of non-sterile formulations for human or animal administration.

10. C
A drug recall in which the use or exposure of the violative substance is not likely to cause adverse health consequences is a Class III recall.

11. C
The USP develops standards regarding the identity, strength, quality, and purity of medications and dietary supplements.

12. B

An oral order for a Schedule II controlled substance is permitted in an emergency situation.

13. C

TJC evaluates and accredits health care organizations and programs in the United States.

14. A

Medications that have no currently accepted medical use and a high potential for abuse are in Schedule I.

15. A

The Food, Drug, and Cosmetic Act of 1938 requires that new drugs must be proven safe and have FDA approval granted prior to marketing.

16. C

The last digit of the DEA number should be 8.

BC372514_
Step 1: Add first, third, and fifth digits: 3 + 2 + 1 = 6
Step 2: Add second, fourth, and sixth digits, then multiply by two: 7 + 5 + 4 = 16 × 2 = 32
Step 3: Add these two answers: 6 + 32 = 38
Step 4: The last digit of this sum will be the last digit of the DEA number.

17. B

A pharmacy is permitted to partially fill a Schedule II controlled substance if the particular medication is out of stock.

18. C

The second segment of an NDC number identifies the strength, dosage form, and formulation of a drug (product code).

19. D

According to federal law, a prescription for a Schedule II controlled substance must be filled within six months of the date written.

20. A

The *United States Pharmacopeia* is a reference book required to be in every pharmacy.

21. C

Chemotherapeutic agents should be prepared in a Class II biological safety cabinet (vertical laminar flow hood).

22. A

The Durham-Humphrey Amendment of 1951 separated drugs into prescription and over-the-counter categories.

23. B

Sublingual nitroglycerin tablets are exempt from the requirements of the Poison Prevention Packaging Act of 1970.

24. D
The first segment of an NDC number identifies the drug manufacturer (labeler).

25. A
If a patient requests that medication be dispensed in a "non-child-resistant" container, the pharmacy should document the information in the patient's record.

26. D
The Comprehensive Drug Abuse Prevention and Control Act of 1970 classified controlled substances into one of five categories based on their abuse potential and accepted medical use.

27. B
The Health Insurance Portability and Accountability Act of 1996 established the provision that all patient medical records and other personal health information must be kept private.

28. A
The Combat Methamphetamine Epidemic Act of 2005 regulates the sale of over-the-counter products containing pseudoephedrine, ephedrine, and phenylpropanolamine.

29. D
The Occupational Safety and Health Act of 1970 sets standards to ensure that employers are providing safe and healthy workplaces, requires that chemical manufacturers provide to the purchaser Safety Data Sheets for hazardous chemicals, and gives employees the right to file a complaint with OSHA regarding safety and health conditions in their workplace.

30. B
iPledge is a Risk Evaluation and Mitigation Strategy (REMS) program that pertains to isotretinoin.

31. B
The Prescription Drug Marketing Act of 1987 prohibits the re-importation of drugs into the United States and regulates the sale of samples.

32. A
Prescriptions for controlled substances may be transferred between pharmacies one time according to federal law.

33. C
The EPA establishes guidelines for the disposal of hazardous waste.

34. D
A forged prescription may be written in different color inks, appear to be photocopied, and the drug prescribed may differ in quantity, directions, or dosage from typical medical usage.

35. D
According to USP <797>, pharmacy personnel who compound low- and medium-risk level sterile products must have their aseptic technique evaluated annually.

36. D
A drug label that does not contain adequate directions for use would be in violation of the Food, Drug, and Cosmetic Act of 1938.

37. C
The Combat Methamphetamine Epidemic Act of 2005 requires that the logbook of pseudoephedrine sales includes product name and quantity, purchaser name and address, and date and time of sale.

38. B
Prescribers must have a DEA number in order to write prescriptions for controlled substances.

39. A
Regarding the over-the-counter sale of select Schedule V medications, the purchaser must complete the Exempt Narcotic Book, no more than one container can be sold to the same purchaser within a 48-hour period, and the product must be sold in the original manufacturer's container.

40. D
No more than five refills are permitted for a Schedule III-V controlled substance prescription.

41. C
DEA Form 222 is used to order Schedule II medications.

42. C
According to federal law, prescriptions for non-controlled medications must initially be filled within six months of the date written.

43. A
Acetaminophen-hydrocodone is an example of a Schedule II controlled substance.

44. C
Regarding the issuance of multiple prescriptions for a particular Schedule II controlled substance from a prescriber to a patient, each prescription must be issued on a separate prescription blank, the prescriber must indicate the earliest date each prescription can be filled, and the issuance of multiple prescriptions must be permitted by applicable state laws.

45. C
Generally, a generic substitution can be made for a drug if the generic product has the same active ingredient(s), dose, dosage form, and route of administration.

46. B
USP <797> provides guidance for the compounding of sterile products.

47. D
Pharmacy records such as prescriptions, controlled substance inventory records, and invoices must be able to be retrieved within 72 hours of a request.

48. A
The federal agency that administers the Medicare and Medicaid programs is the CMS.

49. C
A prescriber who is authorized to prescribe Subutex or Suboxone for the treatment of opioid addiction must have a special DEA number that starts with the letter "X."

50. D
Information on the generic equivalence of drugs can be found in the *Orange Book*.

DOMAIN 3

STERILE AND NON-STERILE COMPOUNDING

QUESTIONS

1. When compounding a pharmaceutical preparation, the prescription should be checked to verify the absence of which of the following?

   a. Dosage errors
   b. Drug interactions
   c. Incompatibilities of ingredients
   d. All of the above

2. Which of the following correctly describes when a laminar flow hood should be turned on?

   a. After compounding activities
   b. Continuously
   c. Immediately before compounding activities
   d. None of the above

3. Which of the following capsule sizes is the smallest?

   a. 000
   b. 0
   c. 1
   d. 5

4. Which of the following is the required air quality for a primary engineering control (PEC)?

   a. ISO Class 1
   b. ISO Class 5
   c. ISO Class 7
   d. ISO Class 8

5. Which of the following references can be used to find the solubility of a drug in a particular solvent when compounding?

   a. American Drug Index
   b. Remington: The Science and Practice of Pharmacy
   c. The Merck Index
   d. Red Book

6. Which of the following types of alcohol is appropriate to use when compounding an oral preparation requiring alcohol?

   a. 70% ethyl alcohol
   b. 70% isopropyl alcohol
   c. 95% ethyl alcohol
   d. Denatured alcohol

7. **When working in a horizontal laminar flow hood, nothing should pass _____ a sterile object.**

   a. behind
   b. in front of
   c. above
   d. below

8. **Which of the following compounding tools is the most appropriate to use when mixing powders?**

   a. Pill tile
   b. Wedgwood mortar
   c. Graduated cylinder
   d. Plastic vial

9. **The process of geometric dilution is necessary to use in which of the following situations?**

   a. The amount of drug relative to the vehicle is small.
   b. The amount of drug relative to the vehicle is large.
   c. The drug has a low potency.
   d. None of the above

10. **Which of the following pieces of personal protective equipment can be reused during the same work shift when an employee leaves a sterile compounding area and later returns?**

   a. Shoe covers
   b. Face mask
   c. Gloves
   d. None of the above

11. **The injection port of an IV bag should be positioned in which of the following directions while compounding in a laminar flow hood?**

   a. Away from the HEPA filter
   b. Towards the HEPA filter
   c. Sideways to the HEPA filter
   d. None of the above

12. **Which of the following are examples of sterile products?**

   a. Parenteral products
   b. Topical products
   c. Oral products
   d. All of the above

13. **According to USP <795>, the beyond-use date for solids and non-aqueous liquids prepared from commercially available dosage forms is _____ in the absence of other data.**

    a. one week
    b. thirty days
    c. ninety days
    d. 25% of the remaining expiration date of the commercial product, or six months, whichever is earlier

14. **When preparing to compound sterile products, personnel must wash their hands and forearms for at least how long?**

    a. Ten seconds
    b. Fifteen seconds
    c. Twenty seconds
    d. Thirty seconds

15. **Alcohol USP refers to which of the following types of alcohol?**

    a. 70% ethyl alcohol
    b. 70% isopropyl alcohol
    c. 95% ethyl alcohol
    d. None of the above

16. **The punch method may be used when compounding which of the following pharmaceutical preparations?**

    a. Suspensions
    b. Solutions
    c. Creams
    d. Capsules

17. **Sterile products are prepared in which of the following areas?**

    a. Ante-area
    b. Buffer area
    c. Primary engineering control (PEC)
    d. All of the above

18. **According to USP <797>, activities such as personnel hand hygiene and garbing procedures, order entry, and product labeling should be performed in which of the following areas?**

    a. Ante-area
    b. Buffer area
    c. Compounding area
    d. None of the above

19. The ability of two liquids to mix in all proportions without separating into two phases is known as _____.

   a. compatibility
   b. solubility
   c. miscibility
   d. stability

20. Which of the following types of water should be used when compounding non-sterile drug preparations according to USP <795>?

   a. Tap water
   b. Chlorinated water
   c. Purified water
   d. Fluorinated water

21. Which of the following types of ingredients should be used for compounding?

   a. Commercially available ingredients
   b. USP or NF grade ingredients
   c. Least expensive ingredients available
   d. Bulk ingredients

22. A _____ filter should be used to sterilize ophthalmic solutions.

   a. 0.22 micron
   b. 0.33 micron
   c. 0.44 micron
   d. 0.55 micron

23. All but which of the following objects should not be placed in a laminar flow hood when compounding?

   a. Pens and pencils
   b. Paper
   c. Labels
   d. Syringes

24. Which of the following needle gauges has the largest diameter?

   a. 13 gauge
   b. 16 gauge
   c. 18 gauge
   d. 20 gauge

25. **Ophthalmic solutions should have which of the following tonicities?**

    a. Hypotonic
    b. Hypertonic
    c. Isotonic
    d. None of the above

26. **Two or more substances that liquefy when mixed at room temperature is referred to as which of the following types of mixture?**

    a. Semisolid
    b. Eutectic
    c. Emulsion
    d. Liquid

27. **To prevent contamination, all manipulations should be performed at least _____ inside a laminar flow hood.**

    a. two inches
    b. four inches
    c. five inches
    d. six inches

28. **Which of the following requires the use of a filter needle?**

    a. Single-dose vials
    b. Multi-dose vials
    c. Ampules
    d. All of the above

29. **How often must ISO Class 5 compounding areas be cleaned?**

    a. Beginning of each work shift
    b. After a spill occurs
    c. When surface contamination is known or suspected
    d. All of the above

30. **Which of the following products is an example of an oleaginous ointment base?**

    a. Velvachol
    b. Aquaphor
    c. Eucerin
    d. White petrolatum

31. Which of the following describes how a laminar flow hood should be cleaned prior to each use?

a. Bottom to top, front to back towards the HEPA filter
b. Top to bottom, back to front away from the HEPA filter
c. Bottom to top, back to front away from the HEPA filter
d. Top to bottom, front to back towards the HEPA filter

32. Which of the following is the correct order of donning personal protective equipment when in the ante-area?

a. Wash hands and forearms, don a non-shedding gown, don shoe covers, don head and facial hair covers, don face mask
b. Don a non-shedding gown, don shoe covers, don head and facial hair covers, don face mask, wash hands and forearms
c. Don shoe covers, don head and facial hair covers, don face mask, wash hands and forearms, don a non-shedding gown
d. Don face mask, don head and facial hair covers, don shoe covers, wash hands and forearms, don a non-shedding gown

33. Which of the following USP chapters describes conditions and practices to prevent harm, including death, to patients that could result from microbial contamination, chemical and physical contaminants, and ingredients of inappropriate quality?

a. USP <795>
b. USP <797>
c. USP <786>
d. USP <1131>

34. Aseptic technique is a method designed to prevent which of the following?

a. Degradation of the product
b. Contamination from microorganisms
c. Incorrect potency of the product
d. Injury to the compounder

35. Which of the following describes how to properly dispose of needles?

a. Discard the needles in a wastebasket.
b. Return the needles to their original packaging.
c. Discard the needles in a puncture-resistant container.
d. None of the above

36. **Pharmacies engaging in compounding activities must keep logs for which of the following?**

    a. Compounding formulas and procedures, but not ingredients purchased
    b. Compounded items
    c. Equipment maintenance records within the past six months only
    d. All of the above

37. **Levigation is a technique used when compounding which of the following dosage forms?**

    a. Suspensions
    b. Suppositories
    c. Capsules
    d. Solutions

38. **Which of the following types of water cannot be used when compounding a sterile preparation?**

    a. Purified water USP
    b. Water for injection USP
    c. Sterile water for injection USP
    d. Bacteriostatic water for injection USP

39. **The air quality of a laminar flow hood should be certified _____.**

    a. every six months
    b. every year
    c. every two years
    d. every three years

40. **USP <797> specifies that radiopharmaceuticals must be compounded using _____.**

    a. properly shielded vials and syringes
    b. ampules
    c. filter needles
    d. 13 gauge needles

41. **Beyond-use dates need to be applied to which of the following types of compounds?**

    a. Non-sterile compounds
    b. Sterile compounds
    c. Topical compounds
    d. All of the above

42. **Which of the following devices should be used when measuring a viscous substance?**

   a. Graduated cylinder
   b. Syringe
   c. Conical cylinder
   d. None of the above

43. **All but which of the following is an example of a type of incompatibility that can occur when compounding IV therapy?**

   a. Phase separation
   b. Miscibility
   c. Turbidity
   d. Precipitate formation

44. **Which of the following ointment bases can take up the most amount of water?**

   a. Eucerin
   b. White petrolatum
   c. Rose water ointment
   d. Aquaphor

45. **All but which of the following are important procedures to follow when using a Class III prescription balance?**

   a. Keep the balance in a locked position when adding or removing weights or materials.
   b. The final measurement can be performed with the cover up.
   c. Weights should not be handled with fingers.
   d. Care should be taken to avoid vibration, dust, moisture, and corrosive vapors.

46. **Which of the following liquid dosage forms always requires shaking before use?**

   a. Solution
   b. Elixir
   c. Tincture
   d. Suspension

47. **The use of a mortar and pestle to reduce particle size is referred to as which of the following?**

   a. Levigation
   b. Sifting
   c. Trituration
   d. Geometric Dilution

48. Which of the following should be included in the verification process for a compounded product?

a. The accuracy of calculations, weights, and measurements
b. Order of mixing of ingredients
c. Appropriate compounding techniques
d. All of the above

49. Which of the following types of water contains antimicrobial agents and can be used for the preparation of parenteral products?

a. Purified water for injection USP
b. Sterile water for injection USP
c. Sterile water for irrigation USP
d. Bacteriostatic water for injection USP

50. All but which of the following bases are commonly used when compounding suppositories?

a. Cocoa butter
b. Hydrogenated vegetable oils
c. Glycerin
d. Cerave

ANSWER KEY

1. D
When compounding a pharmaceutical preparation, the prescription should be checked to verify the absence of dosage errors, drug interactions, and incompatibilities of ingredients.

2. B
A laminar flow hood should be running continuously.

3. D
5 is the smallest capsule size of the choices provided.

4. B
ISO Class 5 is the required air quality for a primary engineering control (PEC).

5. B
Remington: The Science and Practice of Pharmacy can be used to find the solubility of a drug in a particular solvent when compounding.

6. C
95% ethyl alcohol is appropriate to use when compounding an oral preparation requiring alcohol.

7. A
When working in a horizontal laminar flow hood, nothing should pass behind a sterile object.

8. B
A Wedgwood mortar is the appropriate compounding tool to use when mixing powders.

9. A
The process of geometric dilution is necessary to use when the amount of drug relative to the vehicle is small.

10. D
Shoe covers, face masks, and gloves are examples of personal protective equipment that cannot be reused during the same work shift when an employee leaves a sterile compounding area and later returns.

11. B
The injection port of an IV bag should be positioned towards the HEPA filter while compounding in a laminar flow hood.

12. A
Parenteral products are examples of sterile products.

13. D
According to USP <795>, the beyond-use date for solids and non-aqueous liquids prepared from commercially available dosage forms is 25% of the remaining expiration date of the commercial product, or six months, whichever is earlier.

14. D
When preparing to compound sterile products, personnel must wash their hands and forearms for at least thirty seconds.

15. C
Alcohol USP refers to 95% ethyl alcohol.

16. D
The punch method may be used when compounding capsules.

17. C
Sterile products are prepared in a primary engineering control (PEC).

18. A
According to USP <797>, activities such as personnel hand hygiene and garbing procedures, order entry, and product labeling should be performed in the ante-area.

19. C
The ability of two liquids to mix in all proportions without separating into two phases is known as miscibility.

20. C
Purified water should be used when compounding non-sterile drug preparations according to USP <795>.

21. B
USP or NF grade ingredients should be used for compounding.

22. A
A 0.22 micron filter should be used to sterilize ophthalmic solutions.

23. D
Pens and pencils, paper, and labels should not be placed in a laminar flow hood when compounding.

24. A
A 13 gauge needle has the largest diameter of the sizes listed.

25. C
Ophthalmic solutions should be isotonic.

26. B
Two or more substances that liquefy when mixed at room temperature is referred to as a eutectic mixture.

27. D
To prevent contamination, all manipulations should be performed at least six inches inside a laminar flow hood.

28. C
Ampules require the use of a filter needle.

29. D
An ISO Class 5 compounding area must be cleaned at the beginning of each work shift, after a spill occurs, and when surface contamination is known or suspected.

30. D
White petrolatum is an example of an oleaginous ointment base.

31. B
A laminar flow hood should be cleaned top to bottom, back to front away from the HEPA filter prior to each use.

32. C
The correct order of donning personal protective equipment when in the ante-area is: don shoe covers, don head and facial hair covers, don face mask, wash hands and forearms, and don a non-shedding gown.

33. B
USP <797> describes conditions and practices to prevent harm, including death, to patients that could result from microbial contamination, chemical and physical contaminants, and ingredients of inappropriate quality.

34. B
Aseptic technique is a method designed to prevent contamination from microorganisms.

35. C
Needles should be disposed of in a puncture-resistant container.

36. B
Pharmacies engaging in compounding activities must keep logs for compounding formulas and procedures, ingredients purchased, compounded items, and equipment maintenance records.

37. A
Levigation is a technique used when compounding suspensions.

38. A
Purified water USP cannot be used when compounding a sterile preparation.

39. A
The air quality of a laminar flow hood should be certified every six months.

40. A
USP <797> specifies that radiopharmaceuticals must be compounded using properly shielded vials and syringes.

41. D
Beyond-use dates need to be applied to any compounded product.

42. B
A syringe should be used when measuring a viscous substance.

43. B
Phase separation, turbidity, and precipitate formation are examples of incompatibilities that can occur when compounding IV therapy.

44. D
Aquaphor can take up the most amount of water of the choices provided.

45. B
When using a Class III prescription balance, the balance must be kept in a locked position when adding or removing weights or materials, weights should not be handled with fingers, and care should be taken to avoid vibration, dust, moisture, and corrosive vapors.

46. D
A suspension always requires shaking before use.

47. C
The use of a mortar and pestle to reduce particle size is referred to as trituration.

48. D
The accuracy of calculations, weights, and measurements, the order of mixing of ingredients, and appropriate compounding techniques should be included in the verification process for a compounded product.

49. D
Bacteriostatic water for injection USP contains antimicrobial agents and can be used for the preparation of parenteral products.

50. D
Cocoa butter, hydrogenated vegetable oils, and glycerin are bases that are commonly used when compounding suppositories.

DOMAIN 4

MEDICATION SAFETY

QUESTIONS

1. Which of the following is an error-prone abbreviation according to the ISMP?

    a. TPN
    b. QD
    c. NPO
    d. MG

2. Which of the following terms refers to any harm or injury caused by the use of a medication?

    a. Medication allergy
    b. Side effect
    c. Adverse drug event
    d. Precaution

3. Root cause analysis is a method used to _____.

    a. prevent future errors
    b. prevent adverse drug reactions
    c. assess the appropriateness of drug therapy
    d. monitor drug therapy

4. All but which of the following are used to decrease medication errors?

    a. Medication economic analysis
    b. Drug utilization review (DUR)
    c. Medication therapy management (MTM)
    d. Medication reconciliation

5. An organization accredited by The Joint Commission must undergo an on-site survey at least every _____ years.

    a. two
    b. three
    c. four
    d. five

6. Which of the following is an example of a medication error that can occur during the dispensing process?

    a. Selecting the wrong drug formulation
    b. Using inappropriate abbreviations
    c. Inadequately monitoring therapy
    d. Misinterpreting a medication order

7. An error that occurs when something is done incorrectly is classified as which of the following?

a. Systematic error
b. Error of commission
c. Observational error
d. Error of omission

8. The Medicaid Drug Utilization Review (DUR) Program was created by which of the following laws?

a. Food, Drug, and Cosmetic Act of 1938
b. Medicare Prescription Drug Improvement and Modernization Act of 2003
c. Occupational Safety and Health Act of 1970
d. Omnibus Budget Reconciliation Act of 1990

9. Which of the following items are included on The Joint Commission's "Do Not Use" list?

a. U
b. NTG
c. IV
d. BID

10. Which of the following organizations oversees the Medication Error Reporting Program (MERP)?

a. FDA
b. DEA
c. ISMP
d. TJC

11. Medication Guides (MedGuides) are required for which of the following medications?

a. All prescription medications
b. All controlled substance medications
c. Medications that present a serious and significant public health concern
d. All of the above

12. Which of the following processes involves reviewing a patient's complete medication list to avoid inadvertent inconsistencies across transitions of care?

a. Failure mode and effects analysis
b. Root cause analysis
c. Medication reconciliation
d. Drug utilization reviews (DURs)

13. **Which of the following uses a combination of upper and lowercase letters to help distinguish the difference between look-alike and sound-alike medications?**

    a. Bar coding
    b. Tall man lettering
    c. Highlighted lettering
    d. Abbreviation lists

14. **A pharmacy technician is permitted to answer all but which of the following questions regarding a prescription?**

    a. Name of medication
    b. Route of administration
    c. Dosage form
    d. Side effects of the medication

15. **Which of the following is a guideline that identifies potentially harmful and inappropriate medications to use in older adults?**

    a. The Beers List
    b. Medication-Use Evaluation
    c. Clinical Drug Research
    d. Managing Drug Therapy

16. **Mistyping a medication order is an example of an error that can occur during which of the following steps of the medication-use process?**

    a. Dispensing
    b. Transcribing
    c. Prescribing
    d. Monitoring

17. **Which of the following error-reporting programs is an Internet-accessible method that allows hospitals to anonymously report and track errors within their organizations?**

    a. MedMarx
    b. ISMP
    c. MedWatch
    d. MERP

18. **All but which of the following are true regarding a root cause analysis?**

    a. It corrects processes proactively
    b. It is a continuous quality improvement tool
    c. Findings can be used to prevent future errors
    d. It is retrospective

19. **Which of the following regulations encourages the voluntary and confidential reporting of adverse events to improve patient safety?**

    a. Patient Protection Act
    b. Patient Safety and Quality Improvement Act of 2005
    c. Occupational Safety and Health Act of 1970
    d. Food, Drug and Cosmetic Act of 1938

20. **Which of the following medications is associated with a high incidence of medication errors?**

    a. Albuterol
    b. Cyanocobalamin
    c. Insulin
    d. Dexamethasone

21. **Medication therapy management (MTM) is mandated by which of the following?**

    a. Medicare Part C
    b. Medicare Part D
    c. TJC
    d. DEA

22. **Polypharmacy is best described by which of the following?**

    a. Refers to a patient that has a profile at multiple pharmacies
    b. Refers to the use of multiple medications or more than are medically necessary
    c. Refers to a pharmacy that offers multiple services
    d. None of the above

23. **All but which of the following are safe practices regarding the use of crash cart medications?**

    a. Medications should be age-specific
    b. Medications should be in multi-dose vials
    c. Drug expiration dates should be monitored
    d. Medications should be unit-dose

24. **Which of the following strategies can help avoid medication errors?**

    a. Using trailing zeros for whole numbers
    b. Multitasking when processing a prescription
    c. Using a leading zero before a decimal point
    d. Using abbreviations for drug names

25. The Joint Commission requires that before a medication can be removed from an automated dispensing cabinet for a patient, the order must be reviewed by whom (except in emergency situations)?

a. Nurse
b. Physician
c. Pharmacist
d. Pharmacy technician

26. Which of the following activities requires intervention by a pharmacist?

a. Drug utilization reviews (DURs)
b. Labeling prescription bottles
c. Managing inventory
d. Inputting prescription data

27. Which of the following is a database that contains information about adverse events and medication error reports submitted to the FDA?

a. ISMP
b. FAERS
c. TJC
d. VIPPS

28. To decrease medication errors, prescription orders and measurements should use which of the following systems?

a. Apothecary system
b. Avoirdupois system
c. Metric system
d. Imperial system

29. Which of the following are FDA-approved patient handouts that must be dispensed with the original prescription and with each refill for certain medications?

a. Medication information leaflets
b. Package inserts
c. Medication Guides (MedGuides)
d. All of the above

30. Which of the following is a proactive method that analyzes the design of a system to identify where and how it might fail?

a. Root cause analysis
b. Failure mode and effects analysis
c. Data analysis
d. Statistical analysis

31. Which of the following symptoms is a sign that a patient may be experiencing an allergic reaction to a drug?

a. Diarrhea
b. Nausea
c. Drowsiness
d. Rash

32. The Joint Commission requires standard order flow sheets for which of the following classes of medications?

a. Antithrombotics
b. Antibiotics
c. NSAIDs
d. Opioids

33. Patient package inserts are required for which of the following medications?

a. Diuretics
b. Metered-dose inhalers
c. IV medications
d. Steroids

34. Which of the following terms refers to the ongoing review of practitioner prescribing, pharmacist dispensing, and patient use of medication to promote safety?

a. Drug utilization reviews (DURs)
b. Medication Reconciliation
c. Root Cause Analysis
d. Medication Error Reporting Program

35. All but which of the following is a method that should be used to reduce medication errors?

a. Avoid use of error-prone abbreviations
b. Do not use leading zeros
c. Store high-alert medications in a separate area of the pharmacy
d. Use bar code scanners if possible

36. Failing to include information that is necessary for the safe use of a medication is a/an _____.

a. error of commission
b. systematic error
c. random error
d. error of omission

37. **Which of the following programs is mandated under Medicare Part D and promotes the safe and effective use of medications?**

    a. Medication Reconciliation
    b. Drug Utilization Review (DUR) Program
    c. Medication Therapy Management (MTM)
    d. Retrospective Analysis

38. **Which of the following medications are considered high-alert?**

    a. Anticoagulants
    b. Hypoglycemics
    c. Chemotherapeutics
    d. All of the above

39. **According to guidelines developed by the ISMP, maintenance doses of time-critical medications are to be administered within how long of the scheduled time when in an acute care facility?**

    a. Thirty minutes before or after
    b. One hour before or after
    c. Two hours before or after
    d. Three hours before or after

40. **According to the ISMP, all but which of the following dosage forms should never be crushed before administration?**

    a. Extended-release dosage forms
    b. Enteric-coated dosage forms
    c. Slow-release dosage forms
    d. Sugar-coated dosage forms

41. **Which of the following terms refers to a comprehensive medication review that identifies and resolves medication-related problems?**

    a. Medication action plan (MAP)
    b. Medication therapy management (MTM)
    c. Personal medication record (PMR)
    d. Medication administration record (MAR)

42. **The Centers for Medicare and Medicaid Services (CMS) requires which of the following insurance plans to offer MTM services to certain beneficiaries?**

    a. Medicaid
    b. Workers' compensation
    c. TRICARE
    d. Medicare Part D

43. **Which of the following terms refers to the strictest warning put in the labeling of certain prescription drugs by the FDA when there is reasonable evidence of a serious or life-threatening risk?**

    a. Contraindication Warning
    b. FDA Warning
    c. Black Box Warning
    d. Side Effect Warning

44. **Patient profiles should include which of the following in order to increase medication safety?**

    a. Marital status
    b. Drug allergies
    c. Insurance information
    d. Social security number

45. **Which of the following organizations established a voluntary practitioner error reporting program to analyze causes of errors, and shares their findings and recommendations for prevention to healthcare practitioners?**

    a. FDA
    b. TJC
    c. OSHA
    d. ISMP

46. **Which of the following terms refers to the difference between a patient's discharge medication list and the medications they take once at home?**

    a. Medication discrepancy
    b. Medication reconciliation
    c. Medication error
    d. Medication review

47. **Which of the following classes of medication requires a Medication Guide (MedGuide)?**

    a. Thyroid products
    b. Statins
    c. ADHD stimulants
    d. Beta-blockers

48. **All but which of the following can be found on a patient package insert?**

    a. Clinical pharmacology
    b. Precautions
    c. Adverse reactions
    d. Pharmacokinetics

49. Which of the following abbreviations are included on The Joint Commission's "Do Not Use" list?

a. U
b. IU
c. QOD
d. All of the above

50. A patient that misunderstands the instructions for a prescription is an example of an error that can occur during which of the following steps of the medication-use process?

a. Prescribing
b. Monitoring
c. Administration
d. Transcription

ANSWER KEY

1. B
"QD" is an error-prone abbreviation according to the ISMP.

2. C
An adverse drug event refers to any harm or injury caused by the use of a medication.

3. A
Root cause analysis is a method used to prevent future errors.

4. A
Drug utilization review (DUR), medication therapy management (MTM), and medication reconciliation are used to decrease medication errors.

5. B
An organization accredited by The Joint Commission must undergo an on-site survey at least every three years.

6. A
Selecting the wrong drug formulation is an example of a medication error that can occur during the dispensing process.

7. B
An error of commission occurs when something is done incorrectly.

8. D
The Medicaid Drug Utilization Review (DUR) Program was created by the Omnibus Budget Reconciliation Act of 1990.

9. A
"U" is included on The Joint Commission's "Do Not Use" list.

10. C
The ISMP is the organization that oversees the Medication Error Reporting Program (MERP).

11. C
Medication Guides (MedGuides) are required for medications that present a serious and significant public health concern.

12. C
Medication reconciliation involves reviewing a patient's complete medication list to avoid inadvertent inconsistencies across transitions of care.

13. B
Tall man lettering uses a combination of upper and lower case letters to help distinguish the difference between look-alike and sound-alike medications.

14. D
A pharmacy technician is permitted to answer questions regarding the name of medication, route of administration, and the dosage form.

15. A
The Beers List is a guideline that identifies potentially harmful and inappropriate medications to use in older adults.

16. B
Mistyping a medication order is an example of an error that can occur during the transcribing step of the medication-use process.

17. A
MedMarx is an error-reporting program that is an Internet-accessible method that allows hospitals to anonymously report and track errors within their organizations.

18. A
A root cause analysis is a continuous quality improvement tool, findings from the analysis can be used to prevent future errors, and it is retrospective.

19. B
The Patient Safety and Quality Improvement Act of 2005 encourages the voluntary and confidential reporting of adverse events to improve patient safety.

20. C
Insulin is associated with a high incidence of medication errors.

21. B
Medication therapy management (MTM) is mandated by Medicare Part D.

22. B
Polypharmacy refers to the use of multiple medications or more than are medically necessary.

23. B
Using age-specific and unit-dose medications, and monitoring drug expiration dates are safe practices regarding the use of crash cart medications.

24. C
Using a leading zero before a decimal point can help avoid medication errors.

25. C
The Joint Commission requires that before a medication can be removed from an automated dispensing cabinet for a patient, the order must be reviewed by a pharmacist (except in emergency situations).

26. A
Drug utilization reviews (DURs) require intervention by a pharmacist.

27. B
FAERS (FDA Adverse Event Reporting System) is a database that contains information about adverse events and medication error reports submitted to the FDA.

28. C
To decrease medication errors, prescription orders and measurements should use the metric system.

29. C
Medication Guides (MedGuides) are FDA-approved patient handouts that must be dispensed with the original prescription and with each refill for certain medications.

30. B
A failure mode and effects analysis is a proactive method that analyzes the design of a system to identify where and how it might fail.

31. D
A rash is a sign that a patient may be experiencing an allergic reaction to a drug.

32. A
The Joint Commission requires standard order flow sheets for antithrombotics.

33. B
Patient package inserts are required for metered-dose inhalers.

34. A
Drug utilization reviews (DURs) refer to the ongoing review of practitioner prescribing, pharmacist dispensing, and patient use of medication to promote safety.

35. B
Avoiding use of error-prone abbreviations, storing high-alert medications in a separate area of the pharmacy, and using bar code scanners if possible are methods that should be used to reduce medication errors.

36. D
Failing to include information that is necessary for the safe use of a medication is an error of omission.

37. C
Medication therapy management (MTM) is a program mandated under Medicare Part D and promotes the safe and effective use of medications.

38. D
Anticoagulants, hypoglycemics, and chemotherapeutics are medications that are considered high-alert.

39. A
According to guidelines developed by the ISMP, maintenance doses of time-critical medications are to be administered thirty minutes before or thirty minutes after the scheduled time when in an acute care facility.

40. D
According to the ISMP, extended-release, enteric-coated, and slow-release dosage forms should never be crushed before administration.

41. B
Medication therapy management (MTM) refers to a comprehensive medication review that identifies and resolves medication-related problems.

42. D
The Centers for Medicare and Medicaid Services (CMS) requires Medicare Part D insurance plans to offer MTM services to certain beneficiaries.

43. C
A black box warning refers to the strictest warning put in the labeling of certain prescription drugs by the FDA when there is reasonable evidence of a serious or life-threatening risk.

44. B
Patient profiles should include drug allergies in order to increase medication safety.

45. D
The ISMP established a voluntary practitioner error-reporting program to analyze causes of errors, and they share their findings and recommendations for prevention to healthcare practitioners.

46. A
A medication discrepancy refers to the difference between a patient's discharge medication list and the medications they take once at home.

47. C
ADHD stimulants require a Medication Guide (MedGuide).

48. D
Clinical pharmacology, precautions, and adverse reactions can be found on a patient package insert.

49. D
"U", "IU", and "QOD" are included on The Joint Commission's "Do Not Use" list.

50. C
A patient that misunderstands the instructions for a prescription is an example of an error that can occur during the administration step of the medication-use process.

DOMAIN 5

PHARMACY QUALITY ASSURANCE

QUESTIONS

1. Which of the following sets standards for the identity, strength, quality, and purity of medications, dietary supplements, and food ingredients?

    a. United States Pharmacopeia
    b. American Drug Index
    c. Remington: The Science and Practice of Pharmacy
    d. The Merck Manual

2. A laminar flow hood must be turned on for at least _____ before being used.

    a. ten minutes
    b. fifteen minutes
    c. twenty minutes
    d. thirty minutes

3. Which of the following ensures that compounded products are prepared using appropriate procedures?

    a. Quality control
    b. Quality improvement
    c. Quality assurance
    d. Quality management

4. A medication may be recalled for which of the following reasons?

    a. Drug manufacturer goes out of business
    b. Counterfeiting
    c. Generic equivalent becomes available
    d. All of the above

5. Sharps containers are typically which of the following colors?

    a. White
    b. Red
    c. Black
    d. Brown

6. A pharmacy technician must complete _____ of continuing education every two years to maintain certification.

    a. five hours
    b. ten hours
    c. fifteen hours
    d. twenty hours

7. **Which of the following organizations requires pharmacies to maintain SDSs (Safety Data Sheets) for hazardous compounds?**

    a. EPA
    b. FDA
    c. TJC
    d. OSHA

8. **Which of the following types of errors can be reported to MERP?**

    a. Route of administration errors
    b. Wrong drug errors
    c. Drug monitoring errors
    d. All of the above

9. **Which of the following organizations mandates what is addressed in a pharmacy's infection control policy?**

    a. FDA
    b. OSHA
    c. TJC
    d. ISMP

10. **Which of the following types of medication should be counted on a separate tray?**

    a. Diuretics
    b. Oral hypoglycemics
    c. Chemotherapeutic agents
    d. Opioids

11. **Which manner of issuance is preferred for prescriptions to help deter medication errors?**

    a. Verbal
    b. E-prescribing
    c. Fax
    d. Handwritten

12. **Compounds that are prepared within an ISO Class 5 or better environment and do not involve the mixing of more than three commercially manufactured sterile products would be assigned which of the following risk levels?**

    a. Low-risk
    b. Medium-risk
    c. High-risk
    d. Risk levels are not assigned for the compounds described.

13. **Which of the following regulations requires that pharmacists perform a drug utilization review (DUR) when processing a prescription?**

    a. Food, Drug, and Cosmetic Act of 1938
    b. Omnibus Budget Reconciliation Act of 1990
    c. Kefauver-Harris Amendment of 1962
    d. Medicare Prescription Drug, Improvement, and Modernization Act of 2003

14. **Which of the following is true regarding the handling of hazardous drugs?**

    a. Wearing two pairs of gloves is recommended.
    b. Gowns can be reused.
    c. Hazardous drugs can be compounded in any environment.
    d. Spills of hazardous drugs do not need to be cleaned immediately.

15. **The process of _____ can help avoid dosing errors, drug interactions, and therapy duplications.**

    a. dispensing reconciliation
    b. medication reconciliation
    c. automated order entry
    d. point-of-sale reconciliation

16. **Double counting which of the following medications prior to dispensing is a good practice to implement in order to ensure accuracy and safety?**

    a. Anticoagulants
    b. Oral hypoglycemics
    c. Controlled substances
    d. Antibiotics

17. **Which of the following is the FDA's reporting system for adverse drug events?**

    a. MERP
    b. VAERS
    c. MedWatch
    d. ISMP

18. **A pharmacy should do which of the following upon receiving notification of a drug recall?**

    a. Immediately remove the recalled product from the inventory
    b. Destroy the recalled product immediately
    c. Contact the insurance company who received a claim for the recalled product
    d. All of the above

19. Which of the following laws requires the maintenance of a patient profile in any pharmacy setting?

a. Durham-Humphrey Amendment of 1951
b. Omnibus Budget Reconciliation Act of 1990
c. Health Insurance Portability and Accountability Act of 1996
d. Kefauver-Harris Amendment of 1962

20. Which of the following type of syringe should be used when compounding hazardous drugs?

a. Slip-Tip
b. Eccentric
c. Luer-Lok
d. None of the above

21. A Class III prescription balance must be certified _____.

a. every year
b. every two years
c. every three years
d. every five years

22. Which of the following is a record of all the drugs administered to a patient in a facility by a health care professional?

a. POS
b. TAR
c. MAR
d. DUR

23. Which of the following agents should be used to clean counting trays in order to prevent cross-contamination?

a. Methyl alcohol
b. Water
c. Isopropyl alcohol
d. All of the above

24. OSHA mandates that health care workers must be vaccinated for which of the following?

a. Hepatitis A
b. Hepatitis B
c. Tetanus
d. All of the above

25. **Which of the following is true regarding the disposal of used syringes in a sharps container?**

    a. Needles should be recapped.
    b. Needles should be removed from the syringe.
    c. The contents of the sharps container can be pushed down if overfilled.
    d. Syringes should be disposed of with the needle attached.

26. **Which of the following organizations regulates human and veterinary medications, vaccines, biological products, medical devices, and food?**

    a. DEA
    b. EPA
    c. FDA
    d. CMS

27. **HEPA filters in a laminar flow hood remove particles that are at least _____.**

    a. 0.1 microns
    b. 0.2 microns
    c. 0.3 microns
    d. 0.4 microns

28. **All but which of the following is a component of good pharmacy customer service?**

    a. Have a positive attitude
    b. Disregard patient confidentiality
    c. Listen to the customer
    d. Provide accurate information

29. **Which of the following is a post-marketing safety surveillance program that collects information about adverse events that occur after the administration of vaccines licensed in the United States?**

    a. MedWatch
    b. VAERS
    c. FAERS
    d. ISMP

30. **Which of the following codes indicates that a patient requires emergency medical care and is typically in cardiac or respiratory arrest?**

    a. Code Brown
    b. Code Black
    c. Code Orange
    d. Code Blue

31. All but which of the following is considered personal protective equipment?

a. Masks
b. Gowns
c. Gloves
d. Long sleeves

32. Which of the following is used to determine the quality of compounded products by a set of testing activities?

a. Quality management
b. Quality control
c. Quality improvement
d. Quality assurance

33. The USP's drug standards are enforceable in the United States by which of the following organizations?

a. FDA
b. DEA
c. TJC
d. ISMP

34. Microorganisms can be introduced into a laminar flow hood by which of the following?

a. Makeup
b. Jewelry
c. Uncovered facial hair
d. All of the above

35. Hands should be cleaned with soap and water instead of alcohol preparations after caring for a patient with which of the following conditions?

a. Pneumonia
b. Diabetes
c. Influenza
d. Clostridium difficile (C. diff)

36. Compounds that are prepared within an ISO Class 5 or better environment and involve the mixing of more than three commercially manufactured sterile products would be assigned which risk level?

a. Low-risk
b. Medium-risk
c. High-risk
d. Risk levels are not assigned for the compounds described.

37. The Joint Commission accredits all but which of the following organizations?

   a. Long-term care facilities
   b. Doctors' offices
   c. Hospitals
   d. Retail pharmacies

38. Incorrect dosages, drug-disease contraindications, and drug interactions are issues that are addressed by a _____.

   a. MAR
   b. DUR
   c. PAR
   d. MERP

39. Which pharmacy organization oversees pharmacy resources such as the "Do Not Crush List" and "Error-Prone Abbreviations"?

   a. FDA
   b. TJC
   c. ISMP
   d. DEA

40. Which of the following methods should be used if it is necessary to recap a needle?

   a. Two-handed technique
   b. Point needle towards body
   c. One-handed scoop technique
   d. None of the above

41. The use of soap and water is preferred over alcohol-based hand rubs in which of the following scenarios?

   a. Before eating
   b. When hands are visibly soiled
   c. After using the restroom
   d. All of the above

42. Which of the following organizations focuses on medication error prevention and promoting safe medication use?

   a. ISMP
   b. FDA
   c. TJC
   d. OSHA

43. Compounds that are prepared within an environment that is inferior to ISO Class 5 from non-sterile ingredients would be assigned which risk level?

a. Low-risk
b. Medium-risk
c. High-risk
d. Risk levels are not assigned for the compounds described.

44. The process of creating the most accurate list possible of all medications that a patient is taking, and comparing that list to a physician's admission, transfer, and/or discharge orders is referred to as _____.

a. Medication therapy management (MTM)
b. Medication reconciliation
c. Drug utilization review (DUR)
d. Retrospective analysis

45. MERP and VERP are error-reporting programs that are operated by which of the following organizations?

a. FDA
b. DEA
c. ISMP
d. TJC

46. Which of the following techniques should be used when applying alcohol-based hand rubs?

a. Do not rub hands together while rub is drying.
b. Use an adequate amount of rub.
c. Put on gloves before hands are dry.
d. All of the above are correct.

47. Which of the following methods helps to avoid medication errors when filling a prescription?

a. Store sound-alike and look-alike medications in the same area.
b. Compare the NDC numbers on the prescription label to the bulk medication bottle.
c. Store different insulin brands in the same area.
d. Do not compare the prescription label with the original prescription.

48. A complete list of medication recalls can be found on the _____ website.

a. EPA
b. TJC
c. FDA
d. ISMP

49. The distribution of a bulk, sterile vial of an antibiotic into several sterile diluent IV bags is an example of _____ compounding.

a. low-risk
b. medium-risk
c. high-risk
d. no-risk

50. Which of the following drug recall classes is the most severe?

a. Class I
b. Class II
c. Class III
d. Class IV

ANSWER KEY

1. A
The *United States Pharmacopeia* sets standards for the identity, strength, quality, and purity of medications, dietary supplements, and food ingredients.

2. D
A laminar flow hood must be turned on for at least thirty minutes before being used.

3. C
Quality assurance ensures that compounded products are prepared using appropriate procedures.

4. B
A medication may be recalled due to counterfeiting.

5. B
Sharps containers are typically red.

6. D
A pharmacy technician must complete twenty hours of continuing education every two years to maintain certification.

7. D
Pharmacies are required by OSHA to maintain SDSs (Safety Data Sheets) for hazardous compounds.

8. D
Route of administration errors, wrong drug errors, and drug monitoring errors can be reported to MERP.

9. C
The TJC mandates what is addressed in a pharmacy's infection control policy.

10. C
Chemotherapeutic agents should be counted on a separate tray.

11. B
E-prescribing is the preferred manner of issuance for prescriptions to help deter medication errors.

12. A
Compounds that are prepared within an ISO Class 5 or better environment and do not involve the mixing of more than three commercially manufactured sterile products would be assigned a low-risk level.

13. B
The Omnibus Budget Reconciliation Act of 1990 requires that pharmacists perform a drug utilization review (DUR) when processing a prescription.

14. A
Wearing two pairs of gloves is recommended when handling hazardous drugs.

15. B
The process of medication reconciliation can help avoid dosing errors, drug interactions, and therapy duplications.

16. C
Double counting controlled substances prior to dispensing is a good practice to implement in order to ensure accuracy and safety.

17. C
MedWatch is the FDA's reporting system for adverse drug events.

18. A
Upon receiving notification of a drug recall, a pharmacy should immediately remove the recalled product from the inventory, store the recalled product in a separate area, and contact patients who may have received the recalled product.

19. B
The Omnibus Budget Reconciliation Act of 1990 requires the maintenance of a patient profile in any pharmacy setting.

20. C
A Luer-Lok syringe should be used when compounding hazardous drugs.

21. A
A Class III prescription balance must be certified every year.

22. C
A MAR (medication administration record) is a record of all the drugs administered to a patient in a facility by a health care professional.

23. C
Isopropyl alcohol should be used to clean counting trays in order to prevent cross-contamination.

24. B
OSHA mandates that health care workers must be vaccinated for Hepatitis B.

25. D
Syringes should be disposed of with the needle attached in a sharps container.

26. C
The FDA regulates human and veterinary medications, vaccines, biological products, medical devices, and food.

27. C
HEPA filters in a laminar flow hood remove particles that are at least 0.3 microns.

28. B
Having a positive attitude, listening to the customer, and providing accurate information are components of good customer service.

29. B
VAERS (Vaccine Adverse Event Reporting System) is a post-marketing safety surveillance program that collects information about adverse events that occur after the administration of vaccines licensed in the United States.

30. D
Code Blue indicates that a patient requires emergency medical care and is typically in cardiac or respiratory arrest.

31. D
Personal protective equipment includes masks, gowns, and gloves.

32. B
Quality control is used to determine the quality of compounded products by a set of testing activities.

33. A
The USP's drug standards are enforceable in the United States by the FDA.

34. D
Microorganisms can be introduced into a laminar flow hood by makeup, jewelry, and uncovered facial hair.

35. D
Hands should be cleaned with soap and water instead of alcohol preparations after caring for a patient with clostridium difficile (C. diff).

36. B
Compounds that are prepared within an ISO Class 5 or better environment and involve the mixing of more than three commercially manufactured sterile products would be assigned a medium-risk level.

37. D
The Joint Commission accredits long-term care facilities, doctors' offices, and hospitals.

38. B
Incorrect dosages, drug-disease contraindications, and drug interactions are issues that are addressed by a drug utilization review (DUR).

39. C
The ISMP oversees pharmacy resources such as the "Do Not Crush List" and "Error-Prone Abbreviations."

40. C
The one-handed scoop technique should be used if it is necessary to recap a needle.

41. D
The use of soap and water is preferred over alcohol-based hand rubs before eating, when hands are visibly soiled, and after using the restroom.

42. A
The ISMP focuses on medication error prevention and promoting safe medication use.

43. C
Compounds that are prepared within an environment that is inferior to ISO Class 5 from non-sterile ingredients would be assigned a high-risk level.

44. B
The process of creating the most accurate list possible of all medications that a patient is taking, and comparing that list to a physician's admission, transfer, and/or discharge orders is referred to as medication reconciliation.

45. C
MERP and VERP are error-reporting programs that are operated by the ISMP.

46. B
Rubbing hands together until rub dries, using an adequate amount of rub, and not putting on gloves until hands are dry are techniques that should be used when applying alcohol-based hand rubs.

47. B
Comparing the NDC numbers on the prescription label to the bulk medication bottle helps to avoid medication errors when filling a prescription.

48. C
A complete list of medication recalls can be found on the FDA website.

49. B
The distribution of a bulk, sterile vial of an antibiotic into several sterile diluent IV bags is an example of medium-risk compounding.

50. A
Class I recalls are the most severe.

DOMAIN 6

MEDICATION ORDER ENTRY
AND FILL PROCESS

QUESTIONS

1. When billing a third-party provider, which of the following relationship holder codes should be selected for a patient that is the primary cardholder?

    a. 01
    b. 02
    c. 03
    d. 04

2. Translate the following sig into patient directions: i supp pv hs

    a. Insert one suppository rectally at bedtime.
    b. Insert one suppository at bedtime as needed.
    c. Insert one suppository vaginally at bedtime.
    d. Insert one suppository after meals and at bedtime.

3. Which of the following describes the meaning of the root word "card"?

    a. Lung
    b. Kidney
    c. Heart
    d. Skin

4. A "Take with Food" auxiliary label would be appropriate for which of the following types of medications?

    a. Oral corticosteroids
    b. Thyroid medications
    c. Anticoagulants
    d. All of the above

5. Which DAW code should be selected if the prescriber indicates that a generic substitution is permitted but the patient requests the brand product?

    a. DAW 0
    b. DAW 1
    c. DAW 2
    d. DAW 3

6. Pharmacy technicians participate in which of the following tasks?

    a. Providing over-the-counter recommendations
    b. Counseling patients
    c. Processing insurance claims
    d. All of the above

7. **Which of the following medical conditions does a patient have if his/her profile lists the abbreviation "HTN"?**

   a. High blood sugar
   b. Hypertension
   c. Hyperthyroidism
   d. Hypothyroidism

8. **Pharmacy technicians can perform all but which of the following tasks?**

   a. Counting medications
   b. Restocking pharmacy inventory
   c. Counseling patients
   d. Answering the phone

9. **Which of the following medications are not required to be dispensed in child-resistant containers?**

   a. Sublingual nitroglycerin
   b. Oral contraceptives
   c. Inpatient medications
   d. All of the above

10. **Translate the following sig into patient directions: i gtt ou qid**

    a. Instill one drop in each eye four times a day.
    b. Instill one drop in right eye four times a day.
    c. Instill one drop in each ear four times a day.
    d. Instill one drop in left eye four times a day.

11. **The _____ is the part of a prescription that provides instructions for how to take a medication.**

    a. subscription
    b. inscription
    c. superscription
    d. signature (sig)

12. **All but which of the following information is required to be included on an in-patient medication order label?**

    a. Lot number and expiration date of medication
    b. Name and location of patient
    c. Name of medication
    d. Medication manufacturer

13. The _____ is the part of a prescription that indicates the name and dose of the medication to dispense.

    a. inscription
    b. subscription
    c. superscription
    d. signature (sig)

14. Which of the following is the abbreviation for "after meals"?

    a. pc
    b. dtd
    c. ac
    d. prn

15. Which of the following describes the meaning of the root word "gastro"?

    a. Stomach
    b. Kidney
    c. Heart
    d. Lung

16. Which of the following information is required to be included on a sterile product prescription label?

    a. Pharmacy technician's initials
    b. Beyond-use date
    c. Drug manufacturer
    d. Lot number

17. A patient package insert must be provided to patients receiving which of the following medications?

    a. Oral contraceptives
    b. Antibiotics
    c. Statins
    d. Oral hypoglycemics

18. Translate the following sig into patient directions: i gtt as tid x 10d

    a. Instill one drop in right ear three times a day for ten days.
    b. Instill one drop in each ear three times a day for ten days.
    c. Instill one drop in left ear three times a day for ten days.
    d. Instill one drop in left eye three times a day for ten days.

19. **All but which of the following information must be included on a repackaging log?**

    a. Drug manufacturer
    b. Date of repackaging
    c. Pharmacist's initials
    d. Directions for use

20. **An auxiliary label is used to provide which of the following types of supplementary information to a patient?**

    a. Proper administration
    b. Storage requirements
    c. Potential side effects and warnings
    d. All of the above

21. **Which of the following is the abbreviation for "three times a day"?**

    a. qid
    b. qod
    c. tid
    d. bid

22. **Which of the following describes the meaning of the prefix "brady-"?**

    a. Above
    b. Before
    c. Around
    d. Slow

23. **Which of the following information is required to be included on an outpatient prescription label?**

    a. Prescription number
    b. Prescriber's address
    c. Patient's date of birth
    d. Expiration date set by the drug manufacturer

24. **Which of the following describes the meaning of the abbreviation "qod"?**

    a. Every day
    b. Four times a day
    c. Twice a day
    d. Every other day

25. Medications that are sensitive to light should be stored in which of the following types of packaging?

a. Glass bottles
b. Amber containers
c. PVC packaging
d. Hermetic containers

26. Which of the following describes the meaning of the abbreviation "prn"?

a. Per rectum
b. After noon
c. Immediately
d. As needed

27. Containers and administration sets that are made of polyvinyl chloride (PVC) should be avoided with _____.

a. lipid-soluble drugs
b. water-soluble drugs
c. antibiotics
d. emulsions

28. Translate the following sig into patient directions: ii caps po ac and hs

a. Take two capsules by mouth after meals and at bedtime.
b. Take two capsules by mouth before meals and at bedtime.
c. Take two capsules by mouth before meals and after meals.
d. Take two capsules by mouth before breakfast and at bedtime.

29. Which of the following medical conditions does a patient have if his/her profile lists the abbreviation "DM"?

a. Depression
b. Dementia
c. Deep vein thrombosis
d. Diabetes mellitus

30. Which of the following types of insulin should be used in an IV bag?

a. Lente
b. NPH
c. Regular
d. Ultralente

31. Translate the following sig into patient directions: ii caps po bid c̄ food

    a. Take two capsules by mouth twice a day with food.
    b. Take two capsules by mouth three times a day with food.
    c. Take two capsules by mouth four times a day with food.
    d. Take two capsules by mouth once a day with food.

32. The suffix "-algia" refers to which of the following conditions?

    a. Flow or discharge
    b. Fever
    c. Pain
    d. Inflammation

33. Convert the following Roman numeral to an Arabic number: XVI

    a. 4
    b. 6
    c. 14
    d. 16

34. Translate the following sig into patient directions: i tab po tiw

    a. Take one tablet by mouth three times a week.
    b. Take one tablet by mouth three times a day.
    c. Take one tablet by mouth twice a week.
    d. Take one tablet by mouth every week.

35. Which of the following medical conditions does a patient have if his/her profile lists the abbreviation "COPD"?

    a. Congestive heart failure
    b. Chest pain and depression
    c. Chronic obstructive pulmonary disease
    d. Chronic panic disorder

36. Which of the following suffixes refers to a condition of enlargement?

    a. -osis
    b. -megaly
    c. -oma
    d. -itis

37. A "May Cause Drowsiness" auxiliary label would be appropriate for which of the following medications?

    a. Opioid analgesics
    b. Oral corticosteroids
    c. ADHD medications
    d. All of the above

38. Convert the following Roman numeral to an Arabic number: IV

    a. 4
    b. 5
    c. 6
    d. 7

39. When billing a third-party provider, which relationship holder code should be selected for a patient that is the spouse of the primary cardholder?

    a. 01
    b. 02
    c. 03
    d. 04

40. If a prescriber has not indicated on the prescription how many refills are authorized, how many times may the patient have the prescription refilled?

    a. 0
    b. 1
    c. 2
    d. 3

41. Which of the following DAW codes should be selected if the prescriber writes "dispense as written"?

    a. DAW 0
    b. DAW 1
    c. DAW 2
    d. DAW 3

42. Which of the following must a pharmacy technician do if a warning occurs during the drug utilization evaluation phase of processing a prescription?

    a. Enter an override
    b. Alert the pharmacist
    c. Alert the patient
    d. Alert the prescriber

43. Counting trays should be cleaned using isopropyl alcohol after counting which of the following medications?

a. Anticoagulants
b. Thyroid products
c. Oral chemotherapeutics
d. Statins

44. All but which of the following information is commonly included in a patient profile?

a. Patient name and birthdate
b. Health conditions
c. Medication list
d. Social security number

45. Which of the following duties is a pharmacy technician permitted to perform?

a. Taking a new prescription order over the phone
b. Creating a new patient profile
c. Administering immunizations
d. All of the above

46. A prescriber's DEA number is required to be included on a prescription for which of the following types of medications?

a. Injectable medications
b. Controlled substances
c. Chemotherapeutics
d. Oral contraceptives

47. Which of the following information is needed when entering a patient's third-party prescription insurance information?

a. Bank identification number (BIN)
b. Relationship holder code
c. ID number
d. All of the above

48. Which of the following prefixes means "above"?

a. Inter-
b. Hyper-
c. Peri-
d. Trans-

49. A "Shake Well" auxiliary label would be appropriate for which of the following dosage forms?

a. Elixir
b. Solution
c. Suspension
d. Tincture

50. Convert the following Roman numeral to an Arabic number: CXX

a. 25
b. 50
c. 70
d. 120

ANSWER KEY

1. A
When billing a third-party provider, relationship holder code "01" should be selected for a patient that is the primary cardholder.

2. C
The sig "i supp pv hs" translates to "Insert one suppository vaginally at bedtime."

3. C
The meaning of the root word "card" is "heart."

4. A
A "Take with Food" auxiliary label would be appropriate for oral corticosteroids.

5. C
DAW 2 should be selected if the prescriber indicates that a generic substitution is permitted but the patient requests the brand product.

6. C
Pharmacy technicians can participate in processing insurance claims.

7. B
A patient has hypertension if his/her profile lists the abbreviation "HTN."

8. C
Pharmacy technicians can count medications, restock pharmacy inventory, and answer the phone.

9. D
Sublingual nitroglycerin, oral contraceptives, and inpatient medications are not required to be dispensed in child-resistant containers.

10. A
The sig "i gtt ou qid" translates to "Instill one drop in each eye four times a day."

11. D
The signature (sig) is the part of a prescription that provides instructions on how to take a medication.

12. D
The lot number and expiration date of medication, name and location of patient, and name of medication are required to be included on an inpatient medication order label.

13. A
The inscription is the part of a prescription that indicates the name and dose of the medication to dispense.

14. A
The abbreviation for "after meals" is "pc."

15. A
The meaning of the root word "gastro" is "stomach."

16. B
The beyond-use date is required to be included on a sterile product prescription label.

17. A
A patient package insert must be provided to patients receiving oral contraceptives.

18. C
The sig "i gtt as tid x 10d" translates to "Instill one drop in left ear three times a day for ten days."

19. D
A repackaging log must contain the drug manufacturer, date of repackaging, and the pharmacist's initials.

20. D
An auxiliary label is used to provide supplementary information to a patient including the proper administration, storage requirements, and potential side effects and warnings of a medication.

21. C
The abbreviation for "three times a day" is "tid."

22. D
The prefix "brady-" means "slow."

23. A
The prescription number is required to be included on an outpatient prescription label.

24. D
The abbreviation "qod" means "every other day."

25. B
Medications that are sensitive to light should be stored in amber containers.

26. D
The abbreviation "prn" means "as needed."

27. A
Containers and administration sets that are made of polyvinyl chloride (PVC) should be avoided with lipid-soluble drugs.

28. B
The sig "ii caps po ac and hs" translates to "Take two capsules by mouth before meals and at bedtime."

29. D
A patient has diabetes mellitus if his/her profile lists the abbreviation "DM."

30. C
Regular insulin should be used in an IV bag.

31. A
The sig "ii caps po bid c̄ food" translates to "Take two capsules by mouth twice a day with food."

32. C
The suffix "-algia" refers to the condition of pain.

33. D
XVI: X + V + I = 10 + 5 + 1 = 16

34. A
The sig "i tab po tiw" translates to "Take one tablet by mouth three times a week."

35. C
A patient has chronic obstructive pulmonary disease if his/her profile lists the abbreviation "COPD."

36. B
The suffix "-megaly" refers to a condition of enlargement.

37. A
A "May Cause Drowsiness" auxiliary label would be appropriate for opioid analgesics.

38. A
IV: V – I = 5 - 1 = 4

39. B
When billing a third-party provider, the relationship holder code "02" should be selected for a patient that is the spouse of the primary cardholder.

40. A
If a prescriber has not indicated on the prescription how many refills are authorized, the patient cannot have the prescription refilled.

41. B
DAW 1 should be selected if the prescriber writes "dispense as written."

42. B
A pharmacy technician must alert the pharmacist if a warning occurs during the drug utilization evaluation phase of processing a prescription.

43. C
Counting trays should be cleaned using isopropyl alcohol after counting oral chemotherapeutics.

44. D
Patient name and birthdate, health conditions, and a medication list are commonly included in a patient profile.

45. B
A pharmacy technician is permitted to create a new patient profile.

46. B
A prescriber's DEA number is required to be included on a prescription for a controlled substance.

47. D
A bank identification number (BIN), relationship holder code, and ID number are needed when entering a patient's third-party prescription insurance information.

48. B
The prefix "hyper-" means "above."

49. C
A "Shake Well" auxiliary label would be appropriate for a suspension.

50. D
CXX: C + X + X = 100 + 10 + 10 = 120

DOMAIN 7

PHARMACY INVENTORY MANAGEMENT

QUESTIONS

1. **Which of the following are benefits associated with proper inventory management?**

   a. Decreases the cost of ordering medications from wholesalers
   b. Minimizes the occurrence of unexpected stock-outs of products
   c. Prevents costs associated with expiration of inventory
   d. All of the above

2. **Which of the following is true regarding the proper storage of refrigerated medications?**

   a. Pharmacy staff can store food and drinks in the same refrigerator that is used for medications.
   b. Medications can be stored in the refrigerator door.
   c. The temperature of the refrigerator should be monitored twice daily.
   d. All of the above are true.

3. **Which of the following inventory management methods helps to minimize medication costs for a pharmacy?**

   a. Dispensing medications before they expire
   b. Ordering from a preferred wholesaler
   c. Processing returns regularly
   d. All of the above

4. **All but which of the following are important considerations for prescriptions that have not been picked up in a timely manner by a patient?**

   a. They should be restocked for accurate inventory management.
   b. They should be restocked to prevent insurance fraud.
   c. A reminder call to the patient may help minimize the number of unclaimed prescriptions.
   d. They cannot be reused for another patient and should be discarded immediately.

5. **During a controlled substance inventory, an exact count is required for Schedule III, IV, and V substances in packages that are larger than which of the following sizes?**

   a. 100 tablets or capsules
   b. 250 tablets or capsules
   c. 500 tablets or capsules
   d. 1000 tablets or capsules

6. According to federal law, how long must pharmacies keep completed DEA Form 222s on file?

    a. One year
    b. Two years
    c. Three years
    d. Four years

7. Chemotherapy medications are considered to be _____.

    a. hazardous substances
    b. controlled substances
    c. poisonous substances
    d. toxic substances

8. Which of the following is a continually updated list of approved medications for use within a hospital, health care system, or by an insurance company?

    a. Invoice
    b. Purchase order
    c. Formulary
    d. ABC analysis

9. Which of the following inventory management processes refers to ordering products immediately before they are used?

    a. ABC analysis
    b. Last-in-first-out ordering
    c. First-in-first-out ordering
    d. Just-in-time ordering

10. All but which of the following is true regarding beyond-use dates?

    a. They are assigned by the pharmacy.
    b. They are necessary for compounded products.
    c. They are necessary for repackaged medications.
    d. They are assigned by the manufacturer.

11. Which of the following terms refers to the amount of time it takes to use a particular product in the pharmacy inventory in its entirety?

    a. Purchase order
    b. Turnover rate
    c. 80/20 rule
    d. ABC analysis

12. **All but which of the following medications require storage in a separate area of the pharmacy?**

    a. Investigational medications
    b. Expired medications
    c. Recalled medications
    d. Hormone replacement medications

13. **Which of the following inventory management processes refers to setting a maximum and minimum amount of medication that a pharmacy should have in stock, and then having these quantities maintained automatically?**

    a. Just-in-time ordering
    b. PAR (periodic automatic replacement) levels
    c. Last-in-first-out ordering
    d. Maximum and minimum ordering

14. **All but which of the following are important concepts to consider when ordering inventory?**

    a. Product availability
    b. Turnover rate of a medication
    c. Location of manufacturer
    d. Medication expiration date

15. **Which of the following terms refers to the costs of placing an order, receiving goods, and processing payment?**

    a. Turnover rate
    b. Carrying costs
    c. Cost analysis
    d. Procurement costs

16. **Which of the following terms refers to the inventory management strategy that focuses on the top 20% of the items stocked?**

    a. 80/20 ordering
    b. 20% ordering
    c. 20% rule
    d. 80/20 rule

17. **Which of the following terms refers to the inventory management strategy that classifies medications into three classes that are based on their usage and cost?**

    a. PAR (periodic automatic replacement) value
    b. ABC analysis
    c. Economic order quantity
    d. 80/20 rule

18. Which of the following is a list of items that have been delivered to a pharmacy and shows the cost of each item?

a. Purchase order
b. Invoice
c. Perpetual inventory
d. Purchasing report

19. A perpetual inventory is often maintained for which of the following types of medication?

a. Oral chemotherapeutics
b. All controlled substances
c. Hazardous substances
d. Schedule II controlled substances

20. Which of the following steps should be performed when a pharmacy receives a shipment from a wholesaler or manufacturer?

a. Verify that the quantity of boxes or totes delivered matches the expected quantity.
b. Inspect packaging to ensure it has not been tampered with.
c. Inspect items delivered for damage or outdated products.
d. All of the above

21. Which of the following committees of a hospital or managed care organization is responsible for determining which products will be included on a formulary?

a. Health and Wellness Committee
b. Pharmacy and Therapeutics Committee
c. Patient Safety Committee
d. Ethics Committee

22. Which of the following is a form that is used to order medications from a wholesaler?

a. Invoice
b. Purchasing report
c. Purchase order
d. DEA Form 41

23. Which of the following is important to consider when putting a medication order away after it has been delivered?

a. Place the newest stock in front of the old stock.
b. Place the newest stock behind the old stock.
c. Mix the newest stock with the old stock.
d. Discard the old stock.

24. DEA Form 41 must be completed by a pharmacy before which of the following activities can be performed?

a. Ordering controlled substances
b. Dispensing controlled substances
c. Completing a controlled substance inventory
d. Destroying outdated or damaged controlled substances

25. Which of the following may be a reason that a drug manufacturer would recall a product?

a. Product contamination
b. Incorrect labeling
c. Production errors
d. All of the above

26. Which of the following types of formulary allows any medication to be purchased by a hospital or covered by an insurance company?

a. Restricted formulary
b. Open formulary
c. Closed formulary
d. Tiered formulary

27. Which of the following inventory management methods is used to continually monitor the inventory level of a particular product by performing an audit at any given time?

a. Annual inventory counts
b. ABC inventory counts
c. Cycle counts
d. 80/20 counts

28. Which of the following Good Manufacturing Practice (GMP) guidelines should be followed when repackaging medications for use in an inpatient setting?

a. Maintain a repackaging log only for controlled substances.
b. Use appropriate packaging for the medications being repackaged.
c. Have a pharmacy technician verify all medications.
d. All of the above

29. Refrigerator and freezer temperatures should be monitored at least _____ to ensure proper drug storage.

a. once daily
b. twice daily
c. once per week
d. twice per week

30. **Pharmacies that handle hazardous materials must receive and maintain which of the following documents?**

    a. Safety Data Sheets (SDSs)
    b. Package insert
    c. DEA Form 224
    d. Inventory log

31. **Which of the following is a medication that is currently being studied but does not yet have FDA permission to be legally marketed and sold in the United States?**

    a. Off-market drug
    b. Withdrawn drug
    c. Investigational new drug
    d. Recalled drug

32. **Which of the following refers to the costs of keeping items in stock?**

    a. Procurement costs
    b. Acquisition costs
    c. Stock-out costs
    d. Carrying costs

33. **All but which of the following is true regarding the management of crash cart medications?**

    a. The nursing staff is responsible for refilling crash cart medications.
    b. All medications in a tray should be located in the same place each time they are refilled.
    c. Expiration dates of medications should be checked regularly.
    d. Unit-dose packaging is preferred.

34. **A wholesaler is referred to as a _____ when a pharmacy agrees to purchase 80 to 90% of its products from that single wholesaler.**

    a. buying group
    b. prime vendor
    c. pharmacy cooperative
    d. purchasing organization

35. **Which of the following copies of DEA Form 222 must be kept by a pharmacy for its records when ordering Schedule II controlled substances?**

    a. Copy 1
    b. Copy 2
    c. Copy 3
    d. All of the above

36. Which of the following organizations sets the standards for handling and storing chemotherapy, antineoplastic, and cytotoxic agents?

    a. DEA
    b. EPA
    c. FDA
    d. OSHA

37. In a hospital, which of the following areas contains patient-specific medication?

    a. Crash carts
    b. Automated dispensing systems
    c. Floor stock
    d. None of the above

38. Medications that specify in the storage instructions that they are to be kept in a "Dry Place" should not be exposed to humidity exceeding _____ at controlled room temperature.

    a. 40%
    b. 50%
    c. 60%
    d. 70%

39. A master formula for products compounded in a pharmacy must include all but which of the following?

    a. Description of all ingredients and quantities
    b. The beyond-use date of the compounded product
    c. Storage requirements
    d. Pharmacist's name

40. Which of the following terms refers to maintaining a continuous status of the inventory?

    a. Perpetual inventory
    b. Ongoing inventory
    c. Economic inventory
    d. ABC inventory

41. A drug is recalled based on its _____.

    a. product code
    b. lot number and expiration date
    c. package size
    d. date of manufacture

42. **Medications that require storage at room temperature should generally be kept within which of the following temperature ranges?**

    a. 0° and 15°C (32° and 59°F)
    b. 15° and 30°C (59° and 86°F)
    c. 20° and 30°C (68° and 86°F)
    d. 30° and 40°C (86° and 104°F)

43. **Which of the following processes refers to placing newly acquired products behind older products on the shelf?**

    a. Stock rotation
    b. Inventory maintenance
    c. Physical inventory
    d. PAR rotation

44. **A medication that has "05/2018" listed as the expiration date on the manufacturer's container would have an actual expiration date of _____.**

    a. 04/30/2018
    b. 05/01/2018
    c. 05/31/2018
    d. 06/01/2018

45. **During a controlled substance inventory, which of the following classes of medications require an exact count?**

    a. All scheduled medications
    b. Schedule II medications only
    c. Schedule III, IV, and V medications only
    d. Schedule III and IV medications only

46. **Which of the following is a product identifier for all prescription and over-the-counter medications in the United States?**

    a. Lot number
    b. Product number
    c. NDC number
    d. Order code

47. **Medications that bear the label "Protect from Freezing" should not be stored below which of the following temperatures?**

    a. -15°C (5°F)
    b. -10°C (14°F)
    c. -5°C (23°F)
    d. 0°C (32°F)

48. Which of the following types of medications should be treated as hazardous waste?

a. Chemotherapy agents
b. Oral contraceptives
c. Opioid analgesics
d. All of the above

49. A Drug Accountability Record (DAR) must be completed when dispensing which of the following types of medication?

a. Controlled substances
b. Investigational drugs
c. Opioids
d. Thrombolytics

50. All but which of the following is true regarding a pharmacy's inventory turnover rate (ITOR)?

a. As ITOR decreases, sales volume increases.
b. ITOR measures how quickly inventory is purchased, sold, and replaced.
c. ITOR can be increased by increasing sales without increasing inventory.
d. ITOR can be increased by decreasing inventory and maintaining the same sales volume.

ANSWER KEY

1. D
Decreasing the costs of ordering medications from wholesalers, minimizing the occurrence of unexpected stock-outs of products, and preventing costs associated with expiration of inventory are benefits associated with proper inventory management.

2. C
For refrigerated medications, the temperature of the refrigerator should be monitored twice daily.

3. D
Dispensing medications before they expire, ordering from a preferred wholesaler, and processing returns regularly are inventory management methods that help to minimize medication costs for a pharmacy.

4. D
Prescriptions that have not been picked up in a timely manner by a patient should be restocked for accurate inventory management and to prevent insurance fraud. Reminder calls to patients may help minimize the number of unclaimed prescriptions.

5. D
During a controlled substance inventory, an exact count is required for Schedule III, IV, and V substances in packages that are larger than 1000 tablets or capsules.

6. B
Under federal law, pharmacies must keep completed DEA Form 222s on file for two years.

7. A
Chemotherapy medications are considered to be hazardous substances.

8. C
A formulary is a continually updated list of approved medications for use within a hospital, health care system, or by an insurance company.

9. D
Just-in-time ordering is an inventory management process that refers to ordering products immediately before they are used.

10. D
Beyond-use dates are assigned by the pharmacy, are necessary for compounded products, and are necessary for repackaged medications.

11. B
Turnover rate refers to the amount of time it takes to use a particular product in the pharmacy inventory in its entirety.

12. D
Investigational medications, expired medications, and recalled medications require storage in a separate area of the pharmacy.

13. B
PAR (periodic automatic replacement) levels is an inventory management process that refers to setting a maximum and minimum amount of medication that a pharmacy should have in stock, and these quantities are maintained automatically.

14. C
Product availability, the turnover rate of a medication, and a medication's expiration date are important concepts to consider when ordering inventory.

15. D
Procurement costs are the costs of placing an order, receiving goods, and processing payment.

16. D
The 80/20 rule refers to the inventory management strategy that focuses on the top 20% of the items stocked.

17. B
ABC analysis refers to the inventory management strategy that classifies medications into three classes that are based on their usage and cost.

18. B
An invoice is a list of items that have been delivered to a pharmacy and shows the cost of each item.

19. D
A perpetual inventory is often maintained for Schedule II controlled substances.

20. D
Verifying that the quantity of boxes or totes delivered matches the expected quantity, inspecting packaging to ensure it has not been tampered with, and inspecting items delivered for damage or outdated products are steps that should be performed when a pharmacy receives a shipment from a wholesaler or manufacturer.

21. B
The pharmacy and therapeutics committee of a hospital or managed care organization is responsible for determining which products will be included on a formulary.

22. C
A purchase order is a form that is used to order medications from a wholesaler.

23. B
The newest stock should be placed behind the old stock when putting a medication order away after it has been delivered.

24. D
DEA Form 41 must be completed by a pharmacy before an outdated or damaged controlled substance can be destroyed.

25. D
Product contamination, incorrect labeling, and production errors could be reasons that a drug manufacturer would recall a product.

26. B
An open formulary allows any medication to be purchased by a hospital or covered by an insurance company.

27. C
Cycle counts are an inventory management method used to continually monitor the inventory level of a particular product by performing an audit at any given time.

28. B
Using appropriate packaging for the medications being repackaged is a Good Manufacturing Practice (GMP) guideline that should be followed when repackaging medications for use in an inpatient setting.

29. B
Refrigerator and freezer temperatures should be monitored at least twice daily to ensure proper drug storage.

30. A
Pharmacies that handle hazardous materials must receive and maintain safety data sheets (SDSs).

31. C
An investigational new drug is a medication that is currently being studied but does not yet have FDA permission to be legally marketed and sold in the United States.

32. D
Carrying costs refers to the costs of keeping items in stock.

33. A
The pharmacy is responsible for refilling crash cart medications, all medications in a tray should be located in the same place each time they are refilled, the expiration dates of medications in crash carts should be checked regularly, and unit-dose packing is preferred.

34. B
A wholesaler is referred to as a prime vendor when a pharmacy agrees to purchase 80 to 90% of its products from that single wholesaler.

35. C
Copy 3 of DEA Form 222 must be kept by a pharmacy for its records when ordering Schedule II controlled substances.

36. D
OSHA sets the standards for handling and storing chemotherapy, antineoplastic, and cytotoxic agents.

37. D
Crash carts, automated dispensing systems, and floor stock are areas that contain non-patient specific medication in a hospital.

38. A
Medications that specify in the storage instructions that they are to be kept in a "Dry Place" should not be exposed to humidity exceeding 40% at controlled room temperature.

39. D
A master formula for products compounded in a pharmacy must include a description of all ingredients and quantities, the beyond-use date of the compounded product, and storage requirements.

40. A
Perpetual inventory refers to maintaining a continuous status of the inventory.

41. B
A drug is recalled based on its lot number and expiration date.

42. B
Medications that require storage at room temperature should generally be kept within 15° and 30°C (59° and 86°F).

43. A
Stock rotation refers to placing newly acquired products behind older products on the shelf.

44. C
A medication that has "05/2018" listed as the expiration date on the manufacturer's container would have an actual expiration date of 05/31/2018.

45. B
During a controlled substance inventory, all Schedule II medications require an exact count.

46. C
An NDC number is a product identifier for all prescription and over-the-counter medications in the United States.

47. D
Medications that bear the label "Protect from Freezing" should not be stored below 0°C (32°F).

48. A
Chemotherapy agents should be treated as hazardous waste.

49. B
A Drug Accountability Record (DAR) must be completed when dispensing investigational drugs.

50. A
A pharmacy's inventory turnover rate (ITOR) measures how quickly inventory is purchased, sold, and replaced. It can be increased by increasing sales without increasing inventory, and also by decreasing inventory and maintaining the same sales volume.

DOMAIN 8

PHARMACY BILLING AND REIMBURSEMENT

QUESTIONS

1. **Which of the following types of insurance plans are federal programs for patients who are elderly, disabled, receiving dialysis, or low-income?**

   a. Preferred provider organization (PPO)
   b. Workers' compensation
   c. Medicare and Medicaid
   d. Health maintenance organization (HMO)

2. **A prescription drug may require prior authorization from an insurance company in which of the following circumstances?**

   a. It is a medication used for cosmetic purposes.
   b. It is a brand name medication that has a generic available.
   c. It is a medication that is being used at higher than normal doses.
   d. All of the above

3. **Which of the following is an employer-sponsored benefit that allows employees to use pre-tax dollars to pay for eligible health care expenses?**

   a. Capitation account
   b. Fee-for-service account
   c. Flexible spending account (FSA)
   d. Reimbursement account

4. **Which of the following parts of Medicare is a private insurance option that is also known as Medicare Advantage?**

   a. Part A
   b. Part B
   c. Part C
   d. Part D

5. **Which of the following refers to the process that requires a prescriber to obtain approval from a patient's insurance company before a specific medication can be dispensed?**

   a. Initial authorization
   b. Prior authorization
   c. Coordination of benefits
   d. None of the above

6. **Which of the following information is needed by an insurance company when a pharmacy submits a claim for a prescription?**

   a. Lot number of medication
   b. Patient's address
   c. Patient's date of birth
   d. Expiration date of medication

7. **A _____ fee compensates a pharmacy for transferring a drug to the patient, overhead costs, and patient counseling.**

   a. deductible
   b. co-pay
   c. dispensing
   d. capitation

8. **Health care saving plans were created under which of the following laws?**

   a. Omnibus Budget Reconciliation Act of 1990
   b. Health Insurance Portability and Accountability Act of 1996
   c. Kefauver-Harris Amendment of 1962
   d. Medicare Prescription Drug, Improvement, and Modernization Act of 2003

9. **Which of the following refers to the amount of money that must be paid on an annual basis before a co-pay applies?**

   a. Premium
   b. Co-insurance
   c. Deductible
   d. Capitation

10. **In an institutional setting, patients are billed for medications based on information that is provided from which of the following?**

   a. Formulary
   b. Medication Administration Record (MAR)
   c. Pyxis records
   d. Progress notes

11. **Which of the following terms refers to the process of a pharmacy submitting prescription claims to a third-party provider?**

   a. Prior authorization
   b. Adjudication
   c. Coordination of benefits
   d. Remittance advice

12. **The *Red Book* is a resource used to find which of the following?**

    a. Invoice cost
    b. Percent markup
    c. Average wholesale price (AWP)
    d. Net profit

13. **Which of the following parts of Medicare covers doctor visits and outpatient services?**

    a. Part A
    b. Part B
    c. Part C
    d. Part D

14. **All but which of the following statements are true regarding prescription drug plans?**

    a. All prescription drug benefit plans have a deductible.
    b. Some prescription drug plans have a mail-order pharmacy option.
    c. Many prescription drug plans have tiered co-pays.
    d. Employers are not required to provide prescription drug benefits.

15. **Which of the following refers to the average purchase price of a medication at the wholesale level?**

    a. Actual acquisition cost (AAC)
    b. Maximum allowable cost (MAC)
    c. Direct wholesale price (DWP)
    d. None of the above

16. **Which of the following is a unique 10-digit identification number issued to health care providers to transmit health information?**

    a. DEA number
    b. ID number
    c. National Provider Identifier (NPI)
    d. Bank identification number (BIN)

17. **Deductibles for a prescription insurance plan are reset _____.**

    a. every month
    b. every six months
    c. every calendar year
    d. every two years

18. Which of the following parts of Medicare covers certain vaccines that are administered to a patient at a pharmacy?

  a. Part A
  b. Part C
  c. Part D
  d. All of the above

19. All but which of the following strategies are used by pharmacy benefit managers to contain drug costs?

  a. Tiered co-pay structure
  b. Initial co-pay structure
  c. Prior authorizations
  d. Formulary management

20. In which of the following types of insurance plans can a patient choose a primary care physician from a network of providers, and that physician coordinates his/her care?

  a. Health maintenance organization (HMO)
  b. Preferred provider organization (PPO)
  c. Civil labor union
  d. Workers' compensation organization

21. Which of the following types of co-payment arrangement requires a set co-pay regardless of the medication received and its cost?

  a. Percentage co-pay
  b. Multitier co-pay
  c. Variable co-pay
  d. None of the above

22. Which of the following steps should be performed if a "Patient Not Eligible" alert occurs when billing an insurance company for a prescription?

  a. Verify patient's name and date of birth.
  b. Verify the person code.
  c. Check that the correct insurance company is being billed.
  d. All of the above

23. Which of the following refers to the percentage cost that a patient pays for a medication?

  a. Deductible
  b. Co-pay
  c. Tiered formulary
  d. Co-insurance

24. Which of the following describes an alphanumeric number defined by a pharmacy benefit manager that appears on a health insurance card and is used as a secondary identifier for insurance claims?

    a. Bank identification number (BIN)
    b. Member identification number
    c. Processor control number (PCN)
    d. Group number

25. Which of the following parts of Medicare offers prescription drug plans?

    a. Part A
    b. Part B
    c. Part C
    d. Part D

26. Which of the following refers to the coverage gap in Medicare Part D that occurs when the cost of a patient's prescriptions in a given year exceeds a certain amount?

    a. Benefit limitations
    b. Capitation
    c. Stop-loss limit
    d. Donut hole

27. Drug coupon cards for specific medications are provided by _____.

    a. wholesalers
    b. manufacturers
    c. insurance companies
    d. distributors

28. Which of the following is extra health insurance that covers the gap in the Medicare program coverage?

    a. Stop-loss coverage
    b. Health savings account
    c. Flexible savings account
    d. Medigap

29. Which of the following refers to the maximum amount that a plan will pay for generic drugs and brand name drugs that have a generic available?

    a. Suggested wholesale price (SWP)
    b. Average wholesale price (AWP)
    c. Maximum allowable cost (MAC)
    d. Actual acquisition cost (AAC)

30. All but which of the following are examples of government-sponsored health insurance programs?

    a. Medigap
    b. Medicare
    c. Medicaid
    d. TRICARE

31. Which of the following terms refers to the process of determining which insurance coverage should be primary, secondary, etc.?

    a. Remittance advice
    b. Subrogation
    c. Coordination of benefits
    d. Adjudication

32. In which of the following types of insurance plans can a patient visit any doctor without choosing a primary care physician, and pay smaller co-pays for in-network providers but have larger out-of-pocket costs for providers outside of the network?

    a. Health maintenance organization
    b. Government programs
    c. Preferred provider organization
    d. Workers' compensation

33. With a _____ co-payment arrangement, co-pays can change depending on the medication being dispensed.

    a. deductible
    b. variable
    c. percentage
    d. stop-loss

34. Which of the following refers to the act of processing an insurance claim or bill?

    a. Formulary management
    b. Subrogation
    c. Adjudication
    d. Claims adjustment procedure

35. Medicaid covers which of the following groups?

    a. Pregnant women
    b. Employees injured on the job
    c. Individuals above a certain income level
    d. None of the above

36. Which of the following types of insurance is provided by or subsidized by the government?

a. Private insurance
b. Managed care
c. Employer insurance
d. Public insurance

37. Which of the following describes the initial step that should be taken if a "Refill Too Soon" alert occurs when billing an insurance company for a prescription?

a. Verify that the correct days supply was entered.
b. Alert the pharmacist.
c. Call the prescriber.
d. Make the patient pay out-of-pocket for the refill.

38. Which of the following is a six-digit number that appears on a health insurance card and is used to identify a specific plan from a carrier?

a. Member identification number
b. Group number
c. Processor control number (PCN)
d. Bank identification number (BIN)

39. Which of the following parts of Medicare covers nursing care and hospital stays?

a. Part A
b. Part B
c. Part C
d. Part D

40. Which of the following is a preset annual cost that must be paid by a patient before an insurance company will begin paying towards the cost of a prescription?

a. Co-insurance
b. Deductible
c. Co-pay
d. Point-of-sale billing

41. All but which of the following prescribers must have a National Provider Identifier (NPI)?

a. Physicians
b. Nurse practitioners
c. Veterinarians
d. Dentists

42. **Which of the following refers to the amount of money that an individual or business must pay for an insurance plan?**

    a. Deductible
    b. Premium
    c. Capitation
    d. None of the above

43. **Which of the following vendors is responsible for routing prescription information from the pharmacy management software, ensuring that it conforms to NCPDP standards, and routing it to the pharmacy benefit manager?**

    a. Switch vendor
    b. Point-of-sale vendor
    c. Prime vendor
    d. Network vendor

44. **Which of the following refers to the actual cost that a pharmacy paid for a medication?**

    a. Direct price (DP)
    b. Average wholesale price (AWP)
    c. Maximum allowable cost (MAC)
    d. None of the above

45. **Which of the following types of insurance does a consumer receive through his/her employer (or a family member's employer) or through individual purchase?**

    a. Public insurance
    b. Managed care insurance
    c. Private insurance
    d. Hospital insurance

46. **Which of the following is a flat fee that a patient must pay to the pharmacy at the time a medication is dispensed?**

    a. Premium
    b. Co-pay
    c. Co-insurance
    d. Deductible

47. **Medicare covers which of the following groups?**

    a. Senior citizens
    b. Individuals with disabilities
    c. Individuals receiving dialysis
    d. All of the above

48. **Which of the following insurance programs provides benefits for employees who become injured or ill as a direct result of their job?**

   a. Government organizations
   b. Health maintenance organization
   c. Preferred provider organization
   d. Workers' compensation

49. **A National Provider Identifier (NPI) is issued by which of the following organizations?**

   a. TJC
   b. ISMP
   c. CMS
   d. NCPDP

50. **All but which of the following types of information is required by an insurance company when processing a prescription claim?**

   a. Medication expiration date
   b. Patient's name
   c. Patient's identification number
   d. Medication dosage

ANSWER KEY

1. C
Medicare and Medicaid are insurance plans that are federal programs for patients who are elderly, disabled, receiving dialysis, or low-income.

2. D
A prescription drug may require prior authorization from an insurance company if it is a medication used for cosmetic purposes, if it is a brand name medication that has a generic available, or if it is a medication that is being used at higher than normal doses.

3. C
A flexible spending account (FSA) is an employer-sponsored benefit that allows employees to use pre-tax dollars to pay for eligible health care expenses.

4. C
Medicare Part C is a private insurance option that is also known as Medicare Advantage.

5. B
A prior authorization refers to the process that requires a prescriber to obtain approval from a patient's insurance company before a specific medication can be dispensed.

6. C
The patient's date of birth is needed by an insurance company when a pharmacy submits a claim for a prescription.

7. C
A dispensing fee compensates a pharmacy for transferring a drug to the patient, overhead costs, and patient counseling.

8. D
Health care saving plans were created under the Medicare Prescription Drug, Improvement, and Modernization Act of 2003.

9. C
A deductible refers to the amount of money that must be paid on an annual basis before a co-pay applies.

10. B
In an institutional setting, patients are billed for medications based on information that is provided from the medication administration record (MAR).

11. B
Adjudication refers to the process of a pharmacy submitting prescription claims to a third-party provider.

12. C
The *Red Book* is a resource used to find the average wholesale price (AWP).

13. B
Medicare Part B covers doctor visits and outpatient services.

14. A
Some prescription drug plans have a mail-order pharmacy option, and many prescription drug plans have tiered co-pays. Employers are not required to provide prescription drug benefits.

15. D
The average wholesale price (AWP) refers to the average purchase price of a medication at the wholesale level.

16. C
A National Provider Identifier (NPI) is a unique 10-digit identification number issued to health care providers to transmit health information.

17. C
Deductibles for a prescription insurance plan are reset every calendar year.

18. C
Medicare Part D covers certain vaccines that are administered to a patient in a pharmacy.

19. B
A tiered co-pay structure, prior authorizations, and formulary management are strategies used by pharmacy benefit managers to contain drug costs.

20. A
In a health maintenance organization, a patient chooses a primary care physician from a network of providers, and that physician coordinates his/her care.

21. D
A flat rate co-pay requires a set co-pay regardless of the medication received and its cost.

22. D
Verifying a patient's name, date of birth, and person code, and checking that the correct insurance company is being billed are steps that should be performed if a "Patient Not Eligible" alert occurs when billing an insurance company for a prescription.

23. D
Co-insurance refers to the percentage cost that a patient pays for a medication.

24. C
A processor control number (PCN) is an alphanumeric number defined by a pharmacy benefit manager that appears on a health insurance card and is used as a secondary identifier for insurance claims.

25. D
Medicare Part D offers prescription drug plans.

26. D
The "donut hole" refers to the coverage gap in Medicare Part D that occurs when the cost of a patient's prescriptions in a given year exceeds a certain amount.

27. B
Drug coupon cards for specific medications are provided by manufacturers.

28. D
Medigap is extra health insurance that covers the gap in the Medicare program coverage.

29. C
The maximum allowable cost (MAC) refers to the maximum amount that a plan will pay for generic drugs and brand name drugs that have a generic available.

30. A
Medicare, Medicaid, and TRICARE are examples of government sponsored health insurance programs.

31. C
Coordination of benefits refers to the process of determining which insurance coverage should be primary, secondary, etc.

32. C
In a preferred provider organization, a patient can visit any doctor without choosing a primary care physician, and pay smaller co-pays for in-network providers but have larger out-of-pocket costs for providers outside of the network.

33. B
With a variable co-payment arrangement, co-pays can change depending on the medication being dispensed.

34. C
Adjudication refers to the act of processing an insurance claim or bill.

35. A
Medicaid covers pregnant women, individuals with disabilities, and those below a certain income level.

36. D
Public insurance is provided by or subsidized by the government.

37. A
If a "Refill Too Soon" alert occurs when billing an insurance company for a prescription, the initial step that should be taken is to verify that the correct days supply was entered.

38. D
A bank identification number (BIN) is a six-digit number that appears on a health insurance card and is used to identify a specific plan from a carrier.

39. A
Medicare Part A covers nursing care and hospital stays.

40. B
A deductible is a preset annual cost that must be paid by a patient before an insurance company will begin paying towards the cost of a prescription.

41. C
Physicians, nurse practitioners, and dentists have a National Provider Identifier (NPI) in addition to other prescribers.

42. B
The premium refers to the amount of money that an individual or business must pay for an insurance plan.

43. A
A switch vendor is responsible for routing prescription information from the pharmacy management software, ensuring that it conforms to NCPDP standards, and routing it to the pharmacy benefit manager.

44. D
The actual acquisition cost (AAC) refers to the actual cost that a pharmacy paid for a medication.

45. C
Private insurance is the type of insurance that a consumer receives through his/her employer (or a family member's employer) or through individual purchase.

46. B
A co-pay is the flat fee that a patient must pay to the pharmacy at the time a medication is dispensed.

47. D
Medicare covers senior citizens, individuals with disabilities, and those receiving dialysis.

48. D
Workers' compensation is an insurance program that provides benefits for employees who become injured or ill as a direct result of their job.

49. C
A National Provider Identifier (NPI) is issued by the CMS (Centers for Medicare and Medicaid Services).

50. A
The patient's name, identification number, and medication dosage are required by an insurance company when processing a prescription claim.

DOMAIN 9

PHARMACY INFORMATION SYSTEMS USAGE AND APPLICATION

QUESTIONS

1. Which of the following establishes national standards to protect individuals' medical records?

   a. ISMP
   b. NCPDP
   c. HIPAA
   d. MedWatch

2. Computers are commonly used in a pharmacy to perform all but which of the following activities?

   a. Drug utilization evaluations
   b. Drug information reviews
   c. Adverse drug reaction reporting
   d. Manual prescription filling

3. A patient monitoring function that detects a drug-disease interaction would be alerting the user to which of the following issues?

   a. The patient is allergic to the prescribed medication.
   b. The prescribed medication interferes with a medical condition the patient has.
   c. The prescribed medication interferes with another medication the patient is currently taking.
   d. The prescribed medication interferes with a specific laboratory test.

4. Computer database files should be backed up _____.

   a. hourly
   b. daily
   c. weekly
   d. monthly

5. All but which of the following are examples of a computer input device?

   a. Mouse
   b. Keyboard
   c. Microprocessor
   d. Microphone

6. Increasing the speed of preparing medication orders and reducing medication errors are goals of a/an _____.

   a. automated medication system
   b. automated dispensing system
   c. manual medication system
   d. manual dispensing system

7. All but which of the following are true regarding automated decentralized dispensing systems?

a. They are located in patient care units.
b. They provide nurses with ready access to medications.
c. They are located in the central pharmacy.
d. They maintain tight control of drug distribution.

8. Which of the following is an example of computer technology that is used in pharmacies today?

a. Automated dispensing systems
b. Manual tracking systems
c. Biometric coding
d. All of the above

9. Which of the following is true regarding health information technology?

a. Decreases efficiency
b. Decreases communication between healthcare providers
c. Decreases the level of patient care
d. None of the above

10. Which of the following codes are used for billing medication therapy management (MTM) services provided by a pharmacist?

a. ICD-9-CM
b. HCPCS codes
c. CPT codes
d. ICD-10-CM

11. All but which of the following is an example of a biometric identifier?

a. Fingerprints
b. User name and password
c. Iris recognition
d. Face recognition

12. Which of the following allows separate components of a computer system to exchange information?

a. Hardware
b. Processor
c. Software
d. Interface

13. Medications that should not be taken together would be detected in which of the following patient monitoring functions?

a. Drug-food interaction
b. Drug-disease interaction
c. Drug-drug interaction
d. Drug-allergy interaction

14. A computer is commonly used during which of the following steps of prescription processing?

a. Generating labels
b. Billing insurance
c. Inputting customer and prescription data
d. All of the above

15. Information such as patient demographics, progress notes, medications, and medical history can be found in which of the following records?

a. Advanced directives
b. Electronic health care record
c. Medication Administration Record
d. Policy record

16. Which of the following is true regarding e-prescribing?

a. Decreases workflow
b. Eliminates errors due to handwriting
c. Increases data entry
d. All of the above

17. Training all individuals that will be using new technology before implementation is a recommendation provided by which of the following organizations?

a. APhA
b. ISMP
c. TJC
d. PSTAC

18. Which of the following is true regarding accessing a pharmacy's computer system?

a. Unauthorized users should have limited access to the system.
b. It is not necessary for a user to log off each time after using the system.
c. Caution should be used when opening and reading e-mail messages to avoid introducing a virus into the system.
d. All of the above

19. **Which of the following is true regarding the use of bar codes to identify medications in a pharmacy?**

    a. Decreases accuracy when filling orders
    b. Maintains inventory levels
    c. Increases the amount of time it takes to fill an order
    d. All of the above

20. **Computerized pumps are often used in institutional pharmacies to prepare all but which of the following?**

    a. Hyperalimentation solutions
    b. Total parenteral nutrition
    c. The filling of batches of syringes
    d. Unit dose packages

21. **All but which of the following are needed in a patient's medication profile?**

    a. Insurance information
    b. Drug allergies
    c. Birth date
    d. Marital status

22. **A patient monitoring function that detects a therapeutic duplication would be alerting the user to which of the following issues?**

    a. The prescribed medication interferes with a medical condition the patient has.
    b. The prescribed medication interferes with another medication the patient is currently taking.
    c. The prescribed medication is in the same pharmacologic class as another medication the patient is currently taking.
    d. The prescribed medication interferes with a certain food.

23. **Which of the following refers to the various programs used to operate a computer?**

    a. Processor
    b. Interface
    c. Software
    d. Memory

24. **Which the following is true regarding computerized physician order entry?**

    a. System responses are delayed.
    b. Access is available only from the physician's office.
    c. They are not used as a strategy to decrease errors.
    d. Access is available from a variety of settings.

25. **Which of the following is an advantage of an automated centralized dispensing system?**

    a. All systems can accommodate any dosage form, such as injectable or refrigerated items.
    b. Nurses have ready access to medications.
    c. It leads to improved inventory management.
    d. It increases the amount of time pharmacists spend checking orders.

26. **Pharmacies can use technology to perform which of the following tasks?**

    a. Prescription billing
    b. Prescription management
    c. Monitoring medication adherence
    d. All of the above

27. **HIPAA privacy regulations require protecting which of the following forms of protected health information (PHI)?**

    a. Electronic forms only
    b. Electronic and oral forms only
    c. Electronic and paper forms only
    d. Electronic, oral, and paper forms

28. **All but which of the following is an example of a mobile point-of-care device?**

    a. Desktop computer
    b. Tablet
    c. Laptop
    d. Personal digital assistant (PDA)

29. **The NCPDP has developed standards for e-prescribing known as _____.**

    a. MedWatch
    b. ISMP
    c. SCRIPT
    d. VAERS

30. **All but which of the following are examples of automated dispensing systems used in a hospital setting?**

    a. Omnicell
    b. Pyxis
    c. LexisNexis
    d. MedCarousel

31. **All but which of the following are risks of health information technology?**

    a. Implementation may not be carefully planned.
    b. Systems may not be updated consistently.
    c. Efficiency may decrease.
    d. Bar codes may be mislabeled.

32. **Patient records contained in a pharmacy's computer system must be guarded from disclosure, without expressed consent from the patient, to whom?**

    a. Spouse only
    b. Spouse and relative only
    c. Employer and relative only
    d. Spouse, employer, and relative

33. **Which of the following is true regarding automated centralized dispensing systems?**

    a. They can accommodate all dosage forms, such as refrigerated items.
    b. They are located in the central pharmacy.
    c. They provide nurses with ready access to medications.
    d. They cannot be used in unit-dose cart-fill processes.

34. **Which of the following is an example of an automated dispensing system used in retail pharmacies?**

    a. Pyxis
    b. MedCarousel
    c. Omnicell
    d. ScriptPro

35. **Which of the following organizations develops standards for the electronic exchange of healthcare information related to pharmacy services?**

    a. FDA
    b. DEA
    c. CMS
    d. NCPDP

36. **Which of the following is a disadvantage of e-prescribing?**

    a. Decreased efficiency
    b. Pharmacy incurs transaction fees
    c. Decreased access to prescription records
    d. Eliminates errors due to handwriting

37. All but which of the following are true regarding the use of computer systems for inventory management?

a. They can be used to track purchases and the usage of products.
b. They can be used to track outdated medication.
c. They often lead to decreased efficiency compared to manual inventory management.
d. They can be used to update the perpetual inventory of controlled substances.

38. Which of the following is an advantage of automated decentralized dispensing systems?

a. They are located in the central pharmacy.
b. They increase order turnaround time.
c. They provide nurses with ready access to medications.
d. They hinder inventory management.

39. Which of the following is an example of a computer output device?

a. Mouse
b. Keyboard
c. Monitor
d. Microphone

40. Which of the following is contained in a community pharmacy database?

a. Insurance information only
b. Physician files and insurance information only
c. Drug files and physician files only
d. Insurance information, physician files, and drug files

41. Which of the following delivers pharmaceutical care via telecommunications to patients at a remote site?

a. Medication administration record
b. Drug utilization management
c. Telepharmacy
d. E-prescribing

42. Which of the following is an example of an automated dispensing system used to prepare IV admixtures?

a. Pyxis
b. Omnicell
c. Robot-Rx
d. MicroMix

43. All but which of the following are included in the NCPDP standards for e-prescribing?

a. Insurance Processing Standard
b. Billing Unit Standard
c. Prescription Transfer Standard
d. Telecommunication Standard

44. Patient monitoring functions in a computer system can include all but which of the following?

a. Drug-disease interactions
b. Drug-drug interactions
c. Drug-allergy interactions
d. Drug-recall interactions

45. All but which of the following reports are useful to generate using a computer system?

a. Drug use patterns
b. Drug costs
c. Marital status reports
d. Frequency of pharmacist intervention

46. Which of the following is a disadvantage of automation in a pharmacy setting?

a. Decreased efficiency
b. Increased implementation costs
c. Decreased accuracy
d. Increased manual labor

47. Which of the following is a device that allows a computer to transmit data over a network?

a. Processor
b. Modem
c. Plotter
d. Hardware

48. Which of the following is true regarding computerized physician order entry?

a. Does not integrate with electronic medical records
b. Slower transmission to the pharmacy
c. Increases errors compared to handwriting
d. None of the above

49. Which of the following organizations was founded to improve the coding infra-structure used to support the billing of pharmacists' professional services?

    a. TJC
    b. PSTAC
    c. APhA
    d. ISMP

50. Which of the following systems allows a clinician to directly enter medication orders, tests, and procedures into a computer system, which is then transmitted to the pharmacy or appropriate department?

    a. Electronic personal health record
    b. Telepharmacy
    c. Computerized physician order entry
    d. Centralized automation

ANSWER KEY

1. C
HIPAA establishes national standards to protect individuals' medical records.

2. D
Computers are commonly used in a pharmacy to perform activities including drug utilization evaluations, drug information reviews, and adverse drug reaction reporting.

3. B
A patient monitoring function that detects a drug-disease interaction would be alerting the user that the prescribed medication interferes with a medical condition the patient has.

4. B
Computer database files should be backed up daily.

5. C
A mouse, keyboard, and microphone are examples of computer input devices.

6. B
Increasing the speed of preparing medication orders and reducing medication errors are goals of an automated dispensing system.

7. C
Automated decentralized dispensing systems are located in patient care units, they provide nurses with ready access to medications, and they maintain tight control of drug distribution.

8. A
Automated dispensing systems are an example of computer technologies that are used in pharmacies today.

9. D
Increased efficiency, improved communication between healthcare providers, and improved patient care are benefits of health information technology.

10. C
CPT codes are used for billing medication therapy management (MTM) services provided by a pharmacist.

11. B
Fingerprints, iris recognition, and face recognition are examples of biometric identifiers.

12. D
An interface allows separate components of a computer system to exchange information.

13. C
Medications that should not be taken together would be detected in a drug-drug interaction patient monitoring function.

14. D
A computer is commonly used to generate labels, bill insurance, and input customer and prescription data during prescription processing.

15. B
Information such as patient demographics, progress notes, medications, and medical history can be found in an electronic health care record.

16. B
Improving efficiency, eliminating errors due to handwriting, and decreasing data entry are advantages of e-prescribing.

17. C
Training all individuals that will be using new technology before implementation is a recommendation provided by The Joint Commission (TJC).

18. C
Only authorized users should have access to the pharmacy's computer system. It is good practice for a user to log off each time after using the system, and caution should be used when opening and reading e-mail messages to avoid introducing a virus into the system.

19. B
The use of bar codes to identify medications is useful in a pharmacy to increase accuracy when filling orders, to maintain inventory levels, and to save time when filling orders.

20. D
Computerized pumps are often used in institutional pharmacies to prepare hyperalimentation solutions, total parenteral nutrition, and to fill batches of syringes.

21. D
The patient's insurance information, drug allergies, and birth date are needed in a medication profile.

22. C
A patient monitoring function that detects a therapeutic duplication would be alerting the user that the prescribed medication is in the same pharmacologic class as another medication the patient is currently taking.

23. C
Software refers to the various programs used to operate a computer.

24. D
Computerized physician order entry can be accessed from a variety of settings.

25. C
Improved inventory management is an advantage of an automated centralized dispensing system.

26. D
Pharmacies can use technology to perform tasks including prescription billing, prescription management, and monitoring medication adherence.

27. D
HIPAA privacy regulations require protecting electronic, oral, and paper forms of protected health information (PHI).

28. A
A tablet, laptop, and personal digital assistant (PDA) are examples of mobile point-of-care devices.

29. C
The NCPDP has developed standards for e-prescribing known as SCRIPT.

30. C
Omnicell, Pyxis, and MedCarousel are examples of automated dispensing systems used in hospital settings.

31. C
Risks of health information technology include the following: Implementation may not be carefully planned, systems may not be updated consistently, and bar codes may be mislabeled.

32. D
Patient records contained in a pharmacy's computer system must be guarded from disclosure, without expressed consent from the patient, to a patient's spouse, relative and employer.

33. B
Automated centralized dispensing systems are located in the central pharmacy.

34. D
ScriptPro is an example of an automated dispensing system used in retail pharmacies.

35. D
NCPDP develops standards for the electronic exchange of healthcare information related to pharmacy services.

36. B
A disadvantage of e-prescribing is that the pharmacy incurs transaction fees.

37. C
Computer systems can be useful for tracking purchases and usage of products, tracking outdated medication, and updating the perpetual inventory of controlled substances.

38. C
Providing nurses with ready access to medications is an advantage of automated decentralized dispensing systems.

39. C
A monitor is an example of a computer output device.

40. D
Insurance information, physician files, and drug files are contained in a community pharmacy database.

41. C
Telepharmacy delivers pharmaceutical care via telecommunications to patients at a remote site.

42. D
MicroMix is an example of an automated dispensing system used to prepare IV admixtures.

43. A
Billing Unit Standard, Prescription Transfer Standard, and Telecommunication Standard are included in the NCPDP standards for e-prescribing.

44. D
Patient monitoring functions can include drug-disease interactions, drug-drug interactions, and drug-allergy interactions.

45. C
Drug use patterns, drug costs, and frequency of pharmacist intervention are useful reports to generate using a computer system.

46. B
Increased implementation costs can be a disadvantage of automation in a pharmacy setting.

47. B
A modem is a device that allows a computer to transmit data over a network.

48. D
Integration with electronic medical records, faster transmission to the pharmacy, and avoiding errors due to handwriting are advantages of computerized physician order entry.

49. B
The PSTAC was founded to improve the coding infrastructure used to support the billing of pharmacists' professional services.

50. C
Computerized physician order entry is a system that allows a clinician to directly enter medication orders, tests, and procedures into a computer system which is then transmitted to the pharmacy or appropriate department.

PHARMACEUTICAL CALCULATIONS

QUESTIONS

1. A patient is taking 10 milliliters twice daily of amoxicillin 400 mg/5 mL. How many milligrams of amoxicillin is the patient receiving per day?

   a. 800 mg/day
   b. 1600 mg/day
   c. 2200 mg/day
   d. 2400 mg/day

2. A dropper is calibrated to deliver 20 gtts/mL of LCD. How many drops are required for a prescription compound calling for 1.5 milliliters of LCD?

   a. 10 gtts
   b. 15 gtts
   c. 20 gtts
   d. 30 gtts

3. Convert 1:5000 to a percent strength.

   a. 0.02%
   b. 0.2%
   c. 20%
   d. 50%

4. Calculate how many grams each of menthol crystals and camphor crystals are needed for the following prescription:

Menthol crystals	
Camphor crystals	aa 0.5%
Salicylic acid powder	2%
Cerave	qs 120 g

   a. 0.03 g
   b. 0.5 g
   c. 0.6 g
   d. 3 g

5. Amoxicillin 500-mg capsules cost $190.50/500 capsules. How much will a patient be charged for 20 capsules if the pharmacy adds a 35% markup and a $7.00 dispensing fee?

   a. $7.62
   b. $10.29
   c. $14.62
   d. $17.29

6. Convert 1.5 grams to milligrams.

   a. 0.15 mg
   b. 15 mg
   c. 150 mg
   d. 1500 mg

7. A patient is to receive 8 mcg/min of digoxin. The concentration of the digoxin is 1 mg/500 mL of IV fluid. How many milliliters per hour will the patient receive?

   a. 180 mL/hr
   b. 240 mL/hr
   c. 300 mL/hr
   d. 320 mL/hr

8. Calculate the days supply for the following prescription:
Amoxicillin 500 mg, i cap po bid, dispense 14

   a. 3 days
   b. 7 days
   c. 10 days
   d. 14 days

9. One pint of lotion contains 65 milliliters of benzyl alcohol. Calculate the v/v% of benzyl alcohol in the lotion.

   a. 3.1%
   b. 10.2%
   c. 13.7%
   d. 14.8%

10. A physician orders lidocaine 1.5 mg/kg to be given to a patient weighing 165 pounds. The pharmacy has available lidocaine injection in a 4% solution. How many milliliters of the lidocaine solution will be needed for the patient?

   a. 1.92 mL
   b. 2.81 mL
   c. 3.09 mL
   d. 4.76 mL

11. Convert 33 pounds to kilograms.

   a. 9 kg
   b. 15 kg
   c. 21 kg
   d. 72 kg

12. A prescription calls for 0.3 grams of sodium chloride to be dissolved in purified water to form a solution. If the solubility of sodium chloride in water is 1 g/2.8 mL, how many milliliters of water are required to dissolve the sodium chloride?

a. 0.76 mL
b. 0.84 mL
c. 0.97 mL
d. 1.4 mL

13. A pharmacist dissolves 1.25 grams of sucrose in water to make 50 milliliters of solution. What is the percentage of sucrose?

a. 0.25%
b. 0.5%
c. 2.5%
d. 25%

14. The retail price for a blood glucose monitor is $20.99. If the invoice cost is $16.51, what is the markup percentage?

a. 27.1%
b. 28.9%
c. 29.4%
d. 32.5%

15. Convert 76°Fahrenheit to Celsius.

a. 18.6°C
b. 24.4°C
c. 44.3°C
d. 53.2°C

16. A vial of dexamethasone has a concentration of 4 mg/mL. How many milliliters would be given to a patient requiring a 20 milligram dose?

a. 4 mL
b. 5 mL
c. 8 mL
d. 10 mL

17. If 150 milliliters of NS is infused, how many milligrams of sodium chloride will the patient receive?

a. 1200 mg
b. 1350 mg
c. 1420 mg
d. 5100 mg

18. How many teaspoons are in 120 milliliters?

 a. 6 tsp
 b. 8 tsp
 c. 12 tsp
 d. 24 tsp

19. A prescription calls for 200 milliliters of 0.25% prednisolone solution. How many milliliters of 0.5% prednisolone solution are needed to prepare the prescription?

 a. 50 mL
 b. 75 mL
 c. 100 mL
 d. 150 mL

20. What is the body surface area for a patient who weighs 26.4 kg and is 54.1 cm in height?

 a. 0.15 m²
 b. 0.40 m²
 c. 0.63 m²
 d. 0.71 m²

21. 1000 milliliters of fluids must be infused to a patient over six hours. If the calibration of the IV tubing is 10 gtts/mL, how many drops per minute will there be? (round answer to the nearest whole number)

 a. 20 gtts/min
 b. 28 gtts/min
 c. 32 gtts/min
 d. 36 gtts/min

22. Convert 480 milliliters to ounces.

 a. 12 oz
 b. 16 oz
 c. 24 oz
 d. 30 oz

23. A prescription calls for 15 mg/kg of vancomycin every eight hours. How many milligrams of vancomycin will a patient weighing 65 kg receive per day?

 a. 975 mg/day
 b. 1035 mg/day
 c. 2260 mg/day
 d. 2925 mg/day

24. Calculate the days supply for the following prescription:
    Sulfatrim, 1 tsp po q12h, dispense 140 mL

    a. 3 days
    b. 7 days
    c. 10 days
    d. 14 days

25. Calculate how many tablets are needed to fill the following prescription:
    Furosemide 20 mg, ii tabs po bid x 14d

    a. 28 tablets
    b. 42 tablets
    c. 56 tablets
    d. 84 tablets

26. Calculate how many milligrams of enalapril powder are required for the following prescription:

    Enalapril 15 mg/5 mL
    Dispense: 120 mL

    a. 33 mg
    b. 140 mg
    c. 360 mg
    d. 390 mg

27. Calculate how many grams of salicylic acid powder are needed for the following prescription:

    Menthol crystals
    Camphor crystals   aa 0.5%
    Salicylic acid powder   2%
    Cerave   qs 60 g

    a. 0.12 g
    b. 0.3 g
    c. 0.9 g
    d. 1.2 g

28. The package insert for a drug states that 10 milliliters of diluent must be added to 0.25 grams of the dry powder to make a final solution of 100 mg/mL. What is the powder volume?

    a. 2.5 mL
    b. 5 mL
    c. 7.5 mL
    d. 9 mL

29. **Convert 8 fluid ounces to milliliters.**

    a. 80 mL
    b. 120 mL
    c. 240 mL
    d. 300 mL

30. **A wheelchair costs the pharmacy $112.50. If the pharmacy adds a 25% markup to medical equipment, what is the retail price of the wheelchair?**

    a. $128.63
    b. $140.63
    c. $143.54
    d. $147.89

31. **A patient is dispensed a 10 milliliter vial of insulin that contains 100 units/mL. How many days will the vial last if the patient uses 50 units per day?**

    a. 10 days
    b. 18 days
    c. 20 days
    d. 25 days

32. **A prescription calls for 20 mg/kg of a drug for a patient who weighs 70 kilograms. How many milligrams of the drug should the patient receive?**

    a. 800 mg
    b. 1000 mg
    c. 1400 mg
    d. 2100 mg

33. **A prescription calls for cisplatin 50 mg/m^2 per dose. How many milligrams of cisplatin are required for a patient with a BSA of 1.3 m^2?**

    a. 34 mg
    b. 65 mg
    c. 72 mg
    d. 83 mg

34. **Calculate the days supply for the following prescription if 1 milliliter contains 15 drops of medication (round answer down to the nearest whole number): TobraDex Susp, 1 gtt os tid, dispense 2.5 mL bottle**

    a. 10 days
    b. 12 days
    c. 15 days
    d. 20 days

35. **How many 0.5 milliliter doses can be drawn from a 10 milliliter multi-dose vial?**

   a. 5 doses
   b. 10 doses
   c. 20 doses
   d. 25 doses

36. **A patient is to receive 125 mL/hr of an IV bag that is 1 liter. How many hours will the IV bag last?**

   a. 6 hours
   b. 8 hours
   c. 10 hours
   d. 12 hours

37. **How many grams of dextrose are in 250 milliliters of D50W?**

   a. 12.5 g
   b. 50 g
   c. 125 g
   d. 250 g

38. **120 grams of an ointment contains 6 grams of an active ingredient. Calculate the percent strength of the active ingredient in the ointment.**

   a. 0.5%
   b. 4%
   c. 5%
   d. 7.2%

39. **How many milliliters of 30% sucrose can be made from one quart of 70% sucrose?**

   a. 405.4 mL
   b. 1103.7 mL
   c. 2207.3 mL
   d. 2249.3 mL

40. **A TPN order calls for 60 milliequivalents of sodium chloride. Stock vials contain 4 mEq/mL. How many milliliters of sodium chloride should be used?**

   a. 12 mL
   b. 15 mL
   c. 20 mL
   d. 24 mL

41. A patient is to receive 30 units of insulin glargine once daily at bedtime. How many milliliters will be used daily if a 10 milliliter vial contains 100 units/mL?

    a. 0.3 mL
    b. 0.5 mL
    c. 0.7 mL
    d. 1 mL

42. A prescriber orders 1.5 liters of IV fluids to be infused over twelve hours. What is the flow rate in mL/hr?

    a. 110 mL/hr
    b. 125 mL/hr
    c. 187 mL/hr
    d. 210 mL/hr

43. An order is received for 500 milliliters of normal saline to be infused over five hours. If the IV administration set is calibrated to deliver 20 gtts/mL, what will be the flow rate in gtts/min? (round answer to the nearest whole number)

    a. 12 gtts/min
    b. 27 gtts/min
    c. 33 gtts/min
    d. 42 gtts/min

44. Convert 0.25% to a ratio strength.

    a. 1:50
    b. 1:100
    c. 1:200
    d. 1:400

45. Convert 2 grains to milligrams.

    a. 32.5 mg
    b. 64.5 mg
    c. 100 mg
    d. 130 mg

46. A patient is to receive 7 doses of azithromycin 500 mg. If the pharmacy has one gram vials available, how many vials will be needed to prepare the 7 doses?

    a. 2
    b. 3
    c. 4
    d. 6

47. Determine which of the following package sizes is most appropriate to dispense for the following prescription (assume 1 milliliter contains 15 drops of medication): Ciprodex, 4 gtts ad bid x 7d

   a. 2.5 mL
   b. 5 mL
   c. 7.5 mL
   d. 10 mL

48. 20 milliliters of an electrolyte solution and 10 milliliters of a multivitamin solution are added to one liter of NS. If the infusion is to be administered over a period of five hours, what is the flow rate in mL/hr?

   a. 202 mL/hr
   b. 204 mL/hr
   c. 206 mL/hr
   d. 210 mL/hr

49. How many grams each of triamcinolone 0.025% cream and 0.5% cream should be mixed to prepare 60 grams of triamcinolone 0.4% cream?

   a. 10.3 g of triamcinolone 0.025% cream and 49.7 g of triamcinolone 0.5% cream
   b. 12.6 g of triamcinolone 0.025% cream and 47.4 g of triamcinolone 0.5% cream
   c. 17.4 g of triamcinolone 0.025% cream and 42.6 g of triamcinolone 0.5% cream
   d. 18.2 g of triamcinolone 0.025% cream and 41.8 g of triamcinolone 0.5% cream

50. A medication has a wholesale cost of $11.49 and retails for $19.99. The dispensing cost is $2.20. What is the pharmacy's net profit?

   a. $6.30
   b. $8.50
   c. $17.79
   d. $19.99

ANSWER KEY

1. B

$$\frac{10 \text{ mL}}{\text{dose}} \times \frac{2 \text{ doses}}{\text{day}} \times \frac{400 \text{ mg}}{5 \text{ mL}} = 1600 \text{ mg/day}$$

2. D

1.5 mL × 20 gtts/mL = 30 gtts

3. A

Step 1: $\dfrac{1}{5000} = \dfrac{x}{100}$

Step 2: $5000x = 100$

Step 3: $x = 0.02$, therefore the percent strength is 0.02%.

4. C

0.005 × 120 g = 0.6 g

5. D

Step 1: $190.50 ÷ 500 capsules = 0.381 per capsule × 20 capsules = $7.62
Step 2: $7.62 + (7.62 × 35%) = 10.287 + $7.00 = 17.287 = $17.29

6. D

1.5 g × 1000 mg/g = 1500 mg

7. B

Step 1: 8 mcg × 1 mg/1000 mcg = 0.008 mg

Step 2: $\dfrac{0.008 \text{ mg}}{\text{min}} \times \dfrac{500 \text{ mL}}{\text{mg}} \times \dfrac{60 \text{ min}}{\text{hr}} = 240 \text{ mL/hr}$

8. B

14 capsules ÷ 2 capsules per day = 7 days supply

9. C

Step 1: $\dfrac{65 \text{ mL}}{473 \text{ mL}} = \dfrac{x \text{ mL}}{100}$

Step 2: $473x = 6500$

Step 3: $x = 13.7$ mL of benzyl alcohol in 100 mL of lotion, therefore the percentage strength is 13.7%.

10. B

Step 1: 165 lb × 1 kg/2.2 lb = 75 kg

Step 2: 75 kg × 1.5 mg/kg = 112.5 mg ÷ 1000 = 0.1125 g

Step 3: $\dfrac{4 \text{ g}}{100 \text{ mL}} = \dfrac{0.1125 \text{ g}}{x}$

Step 4: $4x = 11.25$

Step 5: $x = 2.81$ mL

11. B

33 lb × 1 kg/2.2 lb = 15 kg

12. B

0.3 g × 2.8 mL/g = 0.84 mL

13. C

Step 1: $\dfrac{1.25 \text{ g}}{50 \text{ mL}} = \dfrac{x}{100}$

Step 2: $50x = 125$

Step 3: $x = 2.5$ g of sucrose in 100 mL of solution, therefore the percentage of sucrose is 2.5%.

14. A

[($20.99 - $16.51)/$16.51] × 100 = 27.1%

15. B

(76 − 32)/1.8 = 24.4°C

16. B

20 mg × 1 mL/4 mg = 5 mL

17. B

Step 1: $\dfrac{0.9 \text{ g}}{100 \text{ mL}} = \dfrac{x \text{ g}}{150 \text{ mL}}$

Step 2: $100x = 135$

Step 3: $x = 1.35$ g × 1000 = 1350 mg

18. D

120 mL × 1 tsp/5 mL = 24 tsp

19. C

Step 1: 0.5% × x mL = 0.25% × 200 mL
Step 2: $0.5x = 50$
Step 3: $x = 100$ mL

20. C

$$\sqrt{\dfrac{(54.1 \text{ cm} \times 26.4 \text{ kg})}{3600}} = 0.63 \text{ m}^2$$

21. B

$\dfrac{1000 \text{ mL}}{6 \text{ hr}} \times \dfrac{\text{hr}}{60 \text{ min}} \times \dfrac{10 \text{ gtts}}{\text{mL}} = 27.8$ gtts/min = 28 gtts/min

22. B

480 mL × 1 oz/30 mL = 16 oz

23. D

Step 1: 65 kg × 15 mg/kg = 975 mg

Step 2: $\dfrac{975 \text{ mg}}{\text{dose}} \times \dfrac{3 \text{ doses}}{\text{day}} = 2925$ mg/day

24. D

$140 \text{ mL} \times \dfrac{\text{dose}}{5 \text{ mL}} \times \dfrac{\text{day}}{2 \text{ doses}} = 14$ days supply

25. C

$\dfrac{2 \text{ tablets}}{\text{dose}} \times \dfrac{2 \text{ doses}}{\text{day}} \times 14$ days = 56 tablets

26. C

120 mL × 15 mg/5 mL = 360 mg

27. D

0.02 × 60 g = 1.2 g

28. C

Step 1: $\dfrac{100 \text{ mg}}{\text{mL}} = \dfrac{250 \text{ mg}}{x \text{ mL}}$

Step 2: $100x = 250$

Step 3: $x = 2.5$ mL

Step 4: 10 mL – 2.5 mL = 7.5 mL

29. C

8 oz × 30 mL/oz = 240 mL

30. B

$112.50 + ($112.50 × 25%) = $140.63

31. C

$10 \text{ mL} \times \dfrac{100 \text{ units}}{\text{mL}} \times \dfrac{\text{day}}{50 \text{ units}} = 20$ days

32. C

70 kg × 20 mg/kg = 1400 mg

33. B

50 mg/m^2 × 1.3 m^2 = 65 mg

34. B

$2.5 \text{ mL} \times \dfrac{15 \text{ gtts}}{\text{mL}} \times \dfrac{\text{day}}{3 \text{ gtts}} = 12.5$ days = 12 days

35. C
10 mL × 1 dose/0.5 mL = 20 doses

36. B
1000 mL × 1 hr/125 mL = 8 hours

37. C
Step 1: $\dfrac{50 \text{ g}}{100 \text{ mL}} = \dfrac{x \text{ g}}{250 \text{ mL}}$

Step 2: $100x = 12{,}500$

Step 3: $x = 125$ g

38. C
Step 1: $\dfrac{6 \text{ g}}{120 \text{ g}} = \dfrac{x \text{ g}}{100}$

Step 2: $120x = 600$

Step 3: $x = 5$ g of active ingredient in 100 g of ointment, therefore the percentage strength is 5%.

39. C
Step 1: 30% × x mL = 70% × 946 mL
Step 2: $30x = 66{,}220$
Step 3: $x = 2207.3$ mL

40. B
60 mEq × 1 mL/4 mEq = 15 mL

41. A
$\dfrac{1 \text{ mL}}{100 \text{ units}} \times \dfrac{30 \text{ units}}{\text{day}} = 0.3$ mL/day

42. B
1500 mL/12 hours = 125 mL/hr

43. C
$\dfrac{500 \text{ mL}}{300 \text{ min}} \times \dfrac{20 \text{ gtts}}{\text{mL}} = 33.3$ gtts/min = 33 gtts/min

44. D
Step 1: $\dfrac{0.25}{100} = \dfrac{1}{x}$

Step 2: $0.25x = 100$

Step 3: $x = 400$, therefore the ratio is 1:400.

45. D
2 gr × 65 mg/gr = 130 mg

46. C
Step 1: 0.5 g × 7 doses = 3.5 g
Step 2: 3.5 g × 1 vial/g = 3.5 vials = 4 vials

47. B
Step 1: $\dfrac{4 \text{ gtts}}{\text{dose}} \times \dfrac{2 \text{ doses}}{\text{day}} \times 7 \text{ days} = 56 \text{ gtts}$

Step 2: 56 gtts × 1 mL/15 gtts = 3.7 mL = 5 mL

48. C
Step 1: 20 mL + 10 mL + 1000 mL = 1030 mL
Step 2: 1030 mL ÷ 5 hr = 206 mL/hr

49. B

Percentage		Parts
0.5%		0.375 parts
	0.4%	
0.025%		0.1 parts
		0.475 total parts

Step 1: Quantity of 0.025% triamcinolone cream: 60 g × 0.1/0.475 = 12.6 g
Step 2: Quantity of 0.5% triamcinolone cream: 60 g × 0.375/0.475 = 47.4 g

50. A
$19.99 – ($11.49 + 2.20) = $6.30

COMPREHENSIVE EXAM 1

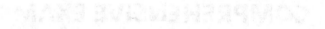

QUESTIONS

1. ACE inhibitors are used in the treatment of all but which of the following conditions?

a. Diabetes
b. Hypertension
c. Asthma
d. Congestive heart failure

2. Which of the following is the abbreviation for "nothing by mouth"?

a. QOD
b. NPO
c. PO
d. TIW

3. Which of the following medications is classified as an antibiotic?

a. Omnicef
b. Lyrica
c. Glucophage
d. Abilify

4. The _____ is the part of the prescription that indicates the quantity of medication to dispense.

a. signature (sig)
b. inscription
c. superscription
d. subscription

5. Calculate how many milliliters per day a patient will use for the following prescription: Lactulose 10 g/15 mL, 2 tbsp po bid x 3d

a. 20 mL
b. 30 mL
c. 60 mL
d. 70 mL

6. All but which of the following medications is used to treat GERD?

a. Prilosec
b. Protonix
c. Nexium
d. Vytorin

7. The sum of acquisition costs, carrying costs, and procurement costs equals which of the following values?

a. Stock-out costs
b. Total costs
c. Net purchases
d. Opportunity costs

8. Which of the following capsule sizes is the largest?

a. 000
b. 00
c. 1
d. 5

9. Which of the following medical conditions does a patient have if his/her profile lists the abbreviation "CHF"?

a. Cardiovascular disease
b. Congestive heart failure
c. Cardiomyopathy
d. Cystic fibrosis

10. Which of the following laws requires that all drug products prepared for commercial distribution must be assigned an NDC number?

a. Pure Food and Drug Act of 1906
b. Prescription Drug Marketing Act of 1987
c. Drug Listing Act of 1972
d. Orphan Drug Act of 1983

11. 125 milliliters of an active ingredient is diluted to one gallon. Calculate the v/v%.

a. 3.3%
b. 4.7%
c. 12.9%
d. 15.1%

12. Which of the following medications is a potassium-sparing diuretic?

a. Spironolactone
b. Diltiazem
c. Furosemide
d. Torsemide

13. Which of the following is the correct order in which drugs are processed by the body?

a. Metabolism, absorption, distribution, excretion
b. Distribution, absorption, metabolism, excretion
c. Absorption, distribution, metabolism, excretion
d. Absorption, metabolism, distribution, excretion

14. Which of the following medications is classified as an opioid?

a. Klonopin
b. Robaxin
c. MS Contin
d. Lyrica

15. Drugs that are marketed in the United States must adhere to standards set by which of the following organizations?

a. USP
b. FDA
c. ISMP
d. TJC

16. Janumet is a combination product containing which of the following diabetes medications?

a. Sitagliptin and metformin
b. Glipizide and metformin
c. Pioglitazone and metformin
d. Glyburide and metformin

17. Which of the following is the mandatory distribution program for isotretinoin?

a. VAERS
b. iPledge
c. VIPPS
d. MedWatch

18. Which of the following is not permitted to be worn in a laminar flow hood?

a. Makeup
b. Latex gloves
c. Eyewear
d. All of the above

19. Medication Guides (MedGuides) address which of the following?

a. Issues that are specific to particular drugs and drug classes
b. Issues that can occur with any FDA-approved medication
c. Issues that can occur with the use of supplements
d. Issues that can occur with the use of over-the-counter medications

20. According to USP <795>, the beyond-use date for solids and non-aqueous liquids prepared from bulk ingredients is _____ in the absence of other data.

a. seven days
b. thirty days
c. ninety days
d. six months

21. Which of the following organizations developed rejection codes to assist in the resolution of declined prescriptions when billing a third-party payer?

a. NCPDP
b. USP
c. FDA
d. TJC

22. Which of the following medications is the generic name for Diovan?

a. Tramadol
b. Valsartan
c. Cephalexin
d. Naproxen

23. An order is received for a heparin infusion with a concentration of 50,000 units/500 mL. The preparation is to be infused at 1000 units/hr. What is the flow rate in mL/hr?

a. 10 mL/hr
b. 30 mL/hr
c. 45 mL/hr
d. 100 mL/hr

24. Which of the following medications is the generic name for Ultracet?

a. Oxycodone-acetaminophen
b. Tramadol
c. Tramadol-acetaminophen
d. Hydrocodone-acetaminophen

25. Which of the following documentation principles promotes the use of performance metrics?

    a. Retrievability
    b. Confidentiality
    c. Auditability
    d. Accuracy

26. All but which of the following medications requires a patient package insert?

    a. Yaz
    b. Lasix
    c. ProAir
    d. Estrace

27. The volume of fluid to be removed from a vial should be replaced with a/an _____ volume of air before withdrawing the fluid to prevent creating a vacuum.

    a. equal
    b. decreasing
    c. smaller
    d. larger

28. Which of the following medications is the generic name for Dyazide?

    a. Valsartan-hydrochlorothiazide
    b. Triamterene-hydrochlorothiazide
    c. Amlodipine-benazepril
    d. Olmesartan-hydrochlorothiazide

29. A maximum of _____ refills can be authorized for a Schedule IV controlled substance prescription.

    a. two
    b. three
    c. five
    d. six

30. PAR (periodic automatic replacement) levels of seasonal medications should be _____ at the beginning of the season to ensure adequate supply.

    a. increased
    b. sharply decreased
    c. gradually decreased
    d. kept the same

31. Which of the following can contribute to the risk of a medication error?

a. Using the avoirdupois system
b. Not using trailing zeros
c. Using leading zeros
d. Using the metric system

32. Which of the following medications is the generic name for Lipitor?

a. Simvastatin
b. Pravastatin
c. Atorvastatin
d. Fluvastatin

33. Which of the following organizations requires that facilities receive and maintain SDSs (Safety Data Sheets) for every hazardous material they stock?

a. DEA
b. FDA
c. OSHA
d. TJC

34. Which of the following is true regarding a prescriber's signature for a handwritten prescription?

a. The signature must be in ink.
b. The signature can be in pencil.
c. The signature can be stamped.
d. None of the above

35. Convert 24.6 kilograms to pounds.

a. 11.2 lb
b. 32.4 lb
c. 54.1 lb
d. 58.3 lb

36. All but which of the following is true regarding the proper use of DEA Form 222?

a. Only one drug may be ordered per line.
b. Mistakes can be crossed out.
c. Only pen or typewriter may be used.
d. Completed forms must be kept on file for two years.

37. **Which of the following medications for osteoporosis is taken once a month?**

    a. Reclast
    b. Fosamax
    c. Boniva
    d. Evista

38. **Which of the following laws allowed the Consumer Product Safety Commission to create standards for child-resistant packaging?**

    a. Comprehensive Drug Abuse Prevention and Control Act of 1970
    b. Poison Prevention Packaging Act of 1970
    c. Durham-Humphrey Amendment of 1951
    d. Pure Food and Drug Act of 1906

39. **Which of the following is required to be included on the label for repackaged medications?**

    a. Name of pharmacy
    b. Directions for use
    c. Lot number of medication
    d. All of the above

40. **What is the body surface area for a patient that weighs 50.9 kg and is 167.6 cm in height?**

    a. 0.98 m²
    b. 1.37 m²
    c. 1.54 m²
    d. 2.37 m²

41. **How many milliliters each of alcohol 91% and alcohol 70% should be mixed to prepare one liter of alcohol 80% solution?**

    a. 491.4 mL of alcohol 70% and 598.6 mL of alcohol 91%
    b. 498.7 mL of alcohol 70% and 501.3 mL of alcohol 91%
    c. 512.3 mL of alcohol 70% and 487.7 mL of alcohol 91%
    d. 523.8 mL of alcohol 70% and 476.2 mL of alcohol 91%

42. **A patient taking metronidazole should avoid which of the following?**

    a. Fish
    b. Alcohol
    c. Dairy products
    d. Bananas

43. Which of the following tablet dosage forms has a special coating that resists stomach acids and is dissolved in the small intestine?

    a. Extended-release tablets
    b. Sublingual tablets
    c. Enteric-coated tablets
    d. Scored tablets

44. Which of the following medications require an "X" DEA number on the prescription?

    a. OxyContin
    b. Vicodin
    c. Suboxone
    d. Adderall

45. When compounding capsules, powders, lozenges, or tablets, the weight of each finished unit should be between _____ of the theoretically calculated weight for each unit.

    a. 80% and 100%
    b. 85% and 100%
    c. 85% and105%
    d. 90% and 110%

46. Which of the following DEA forms must be submitted to document the destruction of outdated or damaged controlled substances?

    a. Form 41
    b. Form 222
    c. Form 225
    d. Form 363

47. Osteoporosis can be treated with all but which of the following medications?

    a. Ibandronate
    b. Raloxifene
    c. Alendronate
    d. Lamotrigine

48. Which of the following is the minimum weighable quantity that can be measured using a Class III prescription balance?

    a. 20 milligrams
    b. 80 milligrams
    c. 100 milligrams
    d. 120 milligrams

49. Calculate how many tablets are needed to fill the following prescription:

Prednisone 10 mg
3 tabs po qd x 3d, 2 tabs po qd x 3d, 1 tab po qd x 3d

a. 10 tablets
b. 15 tablets
c. 18 tablets
d. 20 tablets

50. All but which of the following medications should be taken with food to lessen gastrointestinal side effects?

a. Prednisone
b. Amoxicillin-clavulanate potassium
c. Ibuprofen
d. Levothyroxine

51. A pharmacy may fill a prescription for a Schedule II controlled substance that was faxed from the prescriber in which of the following scenarios?

a. A faxed prescription for a Schedule II controlled substance is never permitted to be filled.
b. The patient lost the original hardcopy prescription.
c. The patient has previously been prescribed the same medication.
d. The patient brings the original hardcopy prescription and it is verified against the fax by the pharmacist at the time of dispensing.

52. Which of the following medications is the generic name for Lopressor?

a. Metoprolol tartrate
b. Fluticasone
c. Metoprolol succinate
d. Levofloxacin

53. How many grams of sodium chloride are in 500 milliliters of normal saline?

a. 4.5 g
b. 5.5 g
c. 6.5 g
d. 9.5 g

54. Which of the following eye drops requires refrigeration prior to opening?

a. Latanoprost
b. Prednisolone
c. Ciprofloxacin
d. Timolol

55. **Which of the following routes of administration is used to deliver a drug systemically through the skin?**

   a. Subcutaneous
   b. Transdermal
   c. Intramuscular
   d. Intravenous

56. **A drug label that is false or misleading would be in violation of which of the following federal laws?**

   a. Pure Food and Drug Act of 1906
   b. Food, Drug, and Cosmetic Act of 1938
   c. Durham-Humphrey Act of 1951
   d. Kefauver-Harris Amendment of 1962

57. **How many tablespoons are in 22.5 milliliters?**

   a. 1.5 tbsp
   b. 2 tbsp
   c. 2.5 tbsp
   d. 4.5 tbsp

58. **All but which of the following medications is used to treat patients with thyroid hormone deficiency?**

   a. Armour Thyroid
   b. Synthroid
   c. Propylthiouracil
   d. Levoxyl

59. **According to federal law, prescriptions for medications in Schedules III-V must initially be filled within _____ of the date written.**

   a. seven days
   b. thirty days
   c. ninety days
   d. six months

60. **Which of the following suffixes refers to inflammation?**

   a. -algia
   b. -ia
   c. -oma
   d. -itis

61. **Which of the following medications is the generic name for Strattera?**

    a. Methylphenidate
    b. Guanfacine
    c. Atomoxetine
    d. Lisdexamfetamine

62. **The dry gum method (continental method) is used to prepare which of the following dosage forms?**

    a. Capsules
    b. Suppositories
    c. Solutions
    d. Emulsions

63. **Which type of measuring device should be used to measure volumes less than 1 milliliter?**

    a. Micropipette
    b. Conical graduate
    c. Cylindrical graduate
    d. Syringe

64. **Convert 1:500 to a percent strength.**

    a. 0.002%
    b. 0.02%
    c. 0.2%
    d. 2%

65. **To maintain sterility while compounding, the _____ of a syringe should never be touched.**

    a. tip
    b. plunger
    c. barrel and plunger
    d. tip and plunger

66. **All but which of the following medications is a cephalosporin antibiotic?**

    a. Omnicef
    b. Zithromax
    c. Keflex
    d. Ceftin

67. **Which of the following medications requires a label stating: "Caution: Federal law prohibits the transfer of this drug to any person other than the patient for whom it was prescribed."**

    a. All prescription medications
    b. Injectable medications
    c. Chemotherapy agents
    d. All controlled substances

68. **Which of the following medications is classified as an SSRI?**

    a. Levetiracetam
    b. Telmisartan
    c. Citalopram
    d. Benzonatate

69. **Which of the following describes the meaning of the abbreviation "NKDA"?**

    a. Known diabetic
    b. No known drug abuse
    c. No known drug allergies
    d. None of the above

70. **Which of the following concentrations of sodium chloride is hypotonic to body cells?**

    a. 0.7% NaCl
    b. 0.9% NaCl
    c. 0.99% NaCl
    d. 1.2% NaCl

71. **How many milliliters of dextrose 50% must be mixed with sterile water to prepare 1.5 liters of dextrose 30% solution?**

    a. 900 mL
    b. 1000 mL
    c. 1200 mL
    d. 2500 mL

72. **Which of the following medications is a fluoroquinolone antibiotic?**

    a. Penicillin
    b. Doxycycline
    c. Ciprofloxacin
    d. Cefdinir

73. The Medicaid Tamper-Resistant Prescription Act requires that all prescriptions for Medicaid beneficiaries be on tamper-resistant paper if the prescription is _____.

    a. faxed
    b. verbal
    c. e-prescribed
    d. handwritten

74. SSRIs are indicated for the treatment of which of the following conditions?

    a. Ulcers
    b. Depression
    c. Hypertension
    d. Gout

75. Which of the following medications should be avoided or used with caution in patients with high blood pressure?

    a. Acetaminophen
    b. Fluticasone
    c. Loratadine
    d. Pseudoephedrine

76. Which of the following needle sizes would be the least likely to cause coring?

    a. 18 gauge
    b. 21 gauge
    c. 23 gauge
    d. 26 gauge

77. Which of the following medications is classified as an antipsychotic?

    a. Sertraline
    b. Clonazepam
    c. Quetiapine
    d. Buspirone

78. All but which of the following is an example of a parenteral dosage form?

    a. Intravenous medications
    b. Intramuscular medications
    c. Subcutaneous medications
    d. Sublingual medications

79. **Prescriptions for Schedule II controlled substances are valid for _____ from the date written.**

    a. thirty days
    b. sixty days
    c. ninety days
    d. six months

80. **Which of the following types of economic analysis studies the perceived benefit of a medication versus its cost?**

    a. Cost-utility analysis
    b. Cost-minimization analysis
    c. Cost-maximization analysis
    d. None of the above

81. **Which of the following medications can decrease a patient's potassium levels?**

    a. Triamterene
    b. Hydrochlorothiazide
    c. Spironolactone
    d. All of the above

82. **Which of the following prefixes means "below"?**

    a. Intra-
    b. Peri-
    c. Hypo-
    d. Brady-

83. **Which of the following is a valid DEA number for a physician named Dr. David Patterson?**

    a. BP8437297
    b. BP8437290
    c. BP8437293
    d. BP8437299

84. **An antipyretic is used to treat which of the following?**

    a. Cough
    b. Fever
    c. Pain
    d. Constipation

85. **Which of the following may indicate that a prescription was not issued for a legitimate medical purpose?**

    a. The patient frequently returns to the pharmacy stating that he/she ran out of medication earlier than expected.
    b. The prescriber writes significantly more prescriptions (or for larger quantities) than what is typical compared to other prescribers in the area.
    c. Individuals who are not regular patrons or live outside the usual geographic area of the pharmacy present prescriptions from the same prescriber.
    d. All of the above

86. **Intramuscular dosage forms should be administered through which of the following methods?**

    a. Injected into a vein
    b. Injected into a muscle
    c. Injected under the skin
    d. Swallowed

87. **Which of the following types of water is used to reconstitute oral products?**

    a. Tap water
    b. Spring water
    c. Purified water USP
    d. Bacteriostatic water

88. **Which of the following products is an example of an absorption ointment base?**

    a. Polybase
    b. Aquaphor
    c. White petrolatum
    d. Rose water ointment

89. **All but which of the following medications is an example of a chemotherapy drug?**

    a. Cyclophosphamide
    b. 5-Fluorouracil
    c. Paclitaxel
    d. Ramipril

90. **Translate the following sig into patient directions: 20 units subq hs**

    a. Inject twenty units under the skin after meals.
    b. Inject twenty units under the skin at bedtime.
    c. Inject twenty units under the skin as needed.
    d. None of the above

91. A patient package insert is required to be provided to patients receiving which of the following medications?

a. Inhalation solutions
b. Topical medications
c. Metered-dose inhalers
d. Injectable medications

92. MAOIs must be avoided with which of the following types of medications?

a. Diuretics
b. SSRIs
c. NSAIDs
d. PDE5 Inhibitors

93. Calculate how many milliliters must be dispensed for the following prescription: Ranitidine 15 mg/mL, i tbsp po bid x 14d

a. 180 mL
b. 210 mL
c. 280 mL
d. 420 mL

94. Proper inventory management is essential for which of the following reasons?

a. To avoid unexpected stock-outs
b. To reduce carrying costs
c. To avoid product loss due to obsolescence
d. All of the above

95. A New Drug Application (NDA) is submitted to which of the following agencies?

a. DEA
b. FDA
c. OSHA
d. TJC

96. The effects of probiotics can be decreased by which of the following types of medication if they are administered at the same time?

a. Diuretics
b. Antibiotics
c. Corticosteroids
d. Antivirals

97. Which of the following medications is the generic name for Bentyl?

a. Diazepam
b. Olmesartan
c. Dicyclomine
d. Carbamazepine

98. Translate the following sig into patient directions: i tab po biw

a. Take one tablet by mouth twice a week.
b. Take one tablet by mouth twice a day.
c. Take one tablet by mouth three times a day.
d. Take one tablet by mouth every two weeks.

99. Which of the following classes of medication relaxes smooth muscle in vascular walls?

a. Proton pump inhibitors
b. Alpha-blockers
c. H2 receptor antagonists
d. Benzodiazepines

100. Which pharmacokinetic phase involves the movement of drug molecules from their site of administration to the blood?

a. Distribution
b. Metabolism
c. Absorption
d. Excretion

ANSWER KEY

1. C
ACE inhibitors are used in the treatment of diabetes, hypertension, and congestive heart failure.

2. B
The abbreviation "NPO" represents "nothing by mouth."

3. A
Omnicef is classified as an antibiotic.

4. D
The subscription is the part of the prescription that indicates the quantity of medication to dispense.

5. C
$$\frac{30 \text{ mL}}{\text{dose}} \times \frac{2 \text{ doses}}{\text{day}} = 60 \text{ mL/day}$$

6. D
Prilosec, Protonix, and Nexium are used to treat GERD.

7. B
The sum of acquisition costs, carrying costs, and procurement costs equals total costs.

8. A
000 is the largest capsule size.

9. B
A patient has congestive heart failure if his/her profile lists the abbreviation "CHF."

10. C
The Drug Listing Act of 1972 requires that all drug products prepared for commercial distribution must be assigned an NDC number.

11. A
Step 1: $\dfrac{125 \text{ mL}}{3785 \text{ mL}} = \dfrac{x \text{ mL}}{100}$

Step 2: $3785x = 12,500$

Step 3: $x = 3.3$ mL of active ingredient in 100 mL of solution, therefore the percentage strength is 3.3%.

12. A
Spironolactone is a potassium-sparing diuretic.

13. C
Absorption, distribution, metabolism, and excretion is the correct order in which drugs are processed by the body.

14. C
MS Contin is classified as an opioid.

15. A
Drugs that are marketed in the United States must adhere to standards set by the USP.

16. A
Janumet is a combination product containing the two diabetes medications sitagliptin and metformin.

17. B
iPledge is the mandatory distribution program for isotretinoin.

18. A
Makeup is not permitted to be worn in a laminar flow hood.

19. A
Medication Guides (MedGuides) address issues that are specific to particular drugs and drug classes.

20. D
According to USP <795>, the beyond-use date for solids and non-aqueous liquids prepared from bulk ingredients is six months in the absence of other data.

21. A
NCPDP is the organization that developed rejection codes that are used when billing a third-party payer.

22. B
Valsartan is the generic name for Diovan.

23. A
$$\frac{500 \text{ mL}}{50{,}000 \text{ units}} \times \frac{1000 \text{ units}}{\text{hr}} = 10 \text{ mL/hr}$$

24. C
Tramadol-acetaminophen is the generic name for Ultracet.

25. C
Auditability is a documentation principle that promotes the use of performance metrics.

26. B
Yaz, ProAir, and Estrace require a patient package insert.

27. A
The volume of fluid to be removed from a vial should be replaced with an equal volume of air before withdrawing the fluid to prevent creating a vacuum.

28. B
Triamterene-hydrochlorothiazide is the generic name for Dyazide.

29. C
A maximum of five refills can be authorized for a Schedule IV controlled substance prescription.

30. A
PAR (periodic automatic replacement) levels of seasonal medications should be increased at the beginning of the season to ensure adequate supply.

31. A
Using the avoirdupois system, using trailing zeros, and not using leading zeros can contribute to the risk of a medication error.

32. C
Atorvastatin is the generic name for Lipitor.

33. C
OSHA requires that facilities receive and maintain SDSs (Safety Data Sheets) for every hazardous material they stock.

34. A
A prescriber's signature for a handwritten prescription must be in ink.

35. C
24.6 kg × 2.2 lb/kg = 54.1 lb

36. B
Only one drug may be ordered per line and only pen or a typewriter may be used to complete DEA Form 222. Pharmacies must keep completed DEA Form 222s on file for two years.

37. C
Boniva is taken once a month.

38. B
The Poison Prevention Packaging Act of 1970 allowed the Consumer Product Safety Commission to create standards for child-resistant packaging.

39. C
The lot number of the medication is required to be included on the label for repackaged medications.

40. C

$$\sqrt{\frac{(167.6 \text{ cm} \times 50.9 \text{ kg})}{3600}} = 1.54 \text{ m}^2$$

41. D

Percentage		Parts
91%		10 parts
	80%	
70%		11 parts
		21 total parts

Step 1: Quantity of 70% alcohol: 1000 mL × 11/21 = 523.8 mL
Step 2: Quantity of 91% alcohol: 1000 mL × 10/21 = 476.2 mL

42. B
A patient taking metronidazole should avoid alcohol.

43. C
Enteric-coated tablets have a special coating that resists stomach acids and is dissolved in the small intestine.

44. C
Suboxone requires an "X" DEA number on the prescription.

45. D
When compounding capsules, powders, lozenges, or tablets, the weight of each finished unit should be between 90% and 110% of the theoretically calculated weight for each unit.

46. A
DEA Form 41 must be submitted to document the destruction of outdated or damaged controlled substances.

47. D
Osteoporosis can be treated with ibandronate, raloxifene, and alendronate.

48. D
120 milligrams is the minimum weighable quantity that can be measured using a Class III prescription balance.

49. C
(3 tabs/day × 3 days) + (2 tabs/day × 3 days) + (1 tab/day × 3 days) = 18 tablets

50. D
Prednisone, amoxicillin-clavulanate potassium, and ibuprofen should be taken with food to lessen gastrointestinal side effects.

51. D
A pharmacy may fill a prescription for a Schedule II controlled substance that was faxed from the prescriber if the patient brings the original hardcopy prescription and it is verified against the fax by the pharmacist at the time of dispensing.

52. A
Metoprolol tartrate is the generic name for Lopressor.

53. A
Step 1: $\dfrac{0.9 \text{ g}}{100 \text{ mL}} = \dfrac{x \text{ g}}{500 \text{ mL}}$

Step 2: $100x = 450$

Step 3: $x = 4.5$ g

54. A
Latanoprost requires refrigeration prior to opening.

55. B
The transdermal route of administration is used to deliver a drug systemically through the skin.

56. B
A drug label that is false or misleading would be in violation of the Food, Drug, and Cosmetic Act of 1938.

57. A
22.5 mL × 1 tbsp/15 mL = 1.5 tbsp

58. C
Armour Thyroid, Synthroid, and Levoxyl are used to treat patients with thyroid hormone deficiency.

59. D
According to federal law, prescriptions for medications in Schedules III-V must initially be filled within six months of the date written.

60. D
The suffix "-itis" refers to inflammation.

61. C
Atomoxetine is the generic name for Strattera.

62. D
The dry gum method (continental method) is used to prepare emulsions.

63. A
A micropipette should be used to measure volumes less than 1 milliliter.

64. C
Step 1: $\dfrac{1}{500} = \dfrac{x}{100}$

Step 2: $500x = 100$

Step 3: $x = 0.2\%$, therefore the percent strength is 0.2%.

65. D
To maintain sterility while compounding, the tip and plunger of a syringe should never be touched.

66. B
Omnicef, Keflex, and Ceftin are cephalosporin antibiotics.

67. D
All controlled substances require a label stating: "Caution: Federal law prohibits the transfer of this drug to any person other than the patient for whom it was prescribed."

68. C
Citalopram is classified as an SSRI.

69. C
The abbreviation "NKDA" represents "no known drug allergies."

70. A
0.7% NaCl is hypotonic to body cells.

71. A
Step 1: $50\% \times x$ mL $= 30\% \times 1500$ mL
Step 2: $50x = 45,000$
Step 3: $x = 900$ mL

72. C
Ciprofloxacin is a fluoroquinolone antibiotic.

73. D
The Medicaid Tamper-Resistant Prescription Act requires that all prescriptions for Medicaid beneficiaries be on tamper-resistant paper if the prescription is handwritten.

74. B
SSRIs are indicated for the treatment of depression.

75. D
Pseudoephedrine should be avoided or used with caution in patients with high blood pressure.

76. D

A 26 gauge needle would be the least likely to cause coring among the needle sizes listed.

77. C

Quetiapine is classified as an antipsychotic.

78. D

Intravenous, intramuscular, and subcutaneous medications are examples of parenteral dosage forms.

79. D

Prescriptions for Schedule II controlled substances are valid for six months from the date written.

80. D

A cost-benefit analysis studies the perceived benefit of a medication versus its cost.

81. B

Hydrochlorothiazide can decrease a patient's potassium levels.

82. C

The prefix "hypo-" means "below."

83. C

BP8437293 is a valid DEA number for physician named Dr. David Patterson.

The last digit of the DEA number should be 3.

BP8437293
Step 1: Add first, third, and fifth digits: 8 + 3 + 2 = 13
Step 2: Add second, fourth, and sixth digits, then multiply by two: 4 + 7 + 9 = 20 × 2 = 40
Step 3: Add these two answers: 13 + 40 = 5<u>3</u>
Step 4: The last digit of this sum will be the last digit of the DEA number.

84. B

An antipyretic is used to treat a fever.

85. D

A prescription may not have been issued for a legitimate medical purpose if the patient frequently returns to the pharmacy stating that he/she ran out of medication earlier than expected, the prescriber writes significantly more prescriptions (or for larger quantities) than what is typical compared to other prescribers in the area, or individuals who are not regular patrons or live outside the usual geographic area of the pharmacy present prescriptions from the same prescriber.

86. B

Intramuscular dosage forms should be injected into a muscle.

87. C
Purified water USP is used to reconstitute oral products.

88. B
Aquaphor is an example of an absorption ointment base.

89. D
Cyclophosphamide, 5-fluorouracil, and paclitaxel are examples of chemotherapy drugs.

90. B
The sig "20 units subq hs" translates to "Inject twenty units under the skin at bedtime."

91. C
A patient package insert is required to be provided to patients receiving metered-dose inhalers.

92. B
MAOIs must be avoided with SSRIs.

93. D
$$\frac{15 \text{ mL}}{\text{dose}} \times \frac{2 \text{ doses}}{\text{day}} \times 14 \text{ days} = 420 \text{ mL}$$

94. D
Proper inventory management is essential to avoid unexpected stock-outs, reduce carrying costs, and to avoid product loss due to obsolescence.

95. B
A New Drug Application (NDA) is submitted to the FDA.

96. B
The effects of probiotics can be decreased by antibiotics if they are administered at the same time.

97. C
Dicyclomine is the generic name for Bentyl.

98. A
The sig "i tab po biw" translates to "Take one tablet by mouth twice a week."

99. B
Alpha-blockers are a class of medications that relax smooth muscle in vascular walls.

100. C
Absorption is the pharmacokinetic phase that involves the movement of drug molecules from their site of administration to the blood.

COMPREHENSIVE EXAM 2

COMPREHENSIVE EXAM 2

QUESTIONS

1. Which of the following medications is the generic name for Lunesta?

a. Zolpidem
b. Levothyroxine
c. Eszopiclone
d. Temazepam

2. Calculate how many capsules need to be dispensed for the following prescription: Vancomycin 125 mg, i cap po q6h x 10d

a. 32
b. 40
c. 54
d. 60

3. Which of the following formularies is comprised of a restricted list of medications selected by a committee, and only certain drugs in each drug class are covered?

a. Tiered formulary
b. Closed formulary
c. Open formulary
d. Restricted formulary

4. Which of the following routes of administration provides the quickest onset?

a. Topical
b. Intramuscular
c. Subcutaneous
d. Intravenous

5. Which of the following is represented by the abbreviation "PO"?

a. By rectum
b. Each eye
c. Right ear
d. By mouth

6. Which of the following medications is the brand name for doxycycline hyclate?

a. Biaxin
b. Namenda
c. Zetia
d. Vibramycin

7. **The amount of solvent required to dissolve a particular amount of drug is referred to as _____.**

    a. miscibility
    b. compatibility
    c. solubility
    d. stability

8. **Which of the following type of purchase occurs when a pharmacy orders a product directly from the manufacturer?**

    a. Point-of-sale purchase
    b. Just-in-time purchase
    c. First-in-first-out purchase
    d. None of the above

9. **Translate the following sig into patient directions: i tab po tid x 7d**

    a. Take one tablet by mouth twice a day for seven days.
    b. Take one tablet by mouth twice a day for seven doses.
    c. Take one tablet by mouth three times a day for seven days.
    d. Take one tablet by mouth four times a day for seven days.

10. **All but which of the following medications is a potassium-sparing diuretic?**

    a. Triamterene
    b. Eplerenone
    c. Hydrochlorothiazide
    d. Spironolactone

11. **A pharmacy that dispenses an investigational new drug is involved in all but which of the following activities?**

    a. Submitting an Investigational New Drug Application
    b. Procurement and storage of the drug
    c. Monitoring and reporting of adverse drug reactions
    d. Patient education

12. **Which of the following describes the meaning of the prefix "peri-"?**

    a. Before
    b. Within
    c. Out
    d. Surrounding

13. Which of the following medications is classified as a hypnotic?

a. Amlodipine
b. Zolpidem
c. Trazodone
d. Lisinopril

14. Personnel hand hygiene and garbing procedures should take place in which of the following areas?

a. Buffer area
b. Clean room
c. Ante-area
d. All of the above

15. Which of the following laws prohibits interstate commerce of misbranded and adulterated food and drugs?

a. Food, Drug, and Cosmetic Act of 1938
b. Kefauver-Harris Amendment of 1962
c. Pure Food and Drug Act of 1906
d. Prescription Drug Marketing Act of 1987

16. Which of the following medications is the brand name for fenofibrate?

a. TriCor
b. Levaquin
c. Zetia
d. Vistaril

17. Convert 75 micrograms to milligrams.

a. 0.0075 mg
b. 0.075 mg
c. 0.75 mg
d. 750 mg

18. All but which of the following statements is true regarding the Combat Meth-amphetamine Epidemic Act of 2005?

a. It applies to both prescription and nonprescription drug products containing ephedrine, pseudoephedrine, and phenylpropanolamine.
b. Regulated products must be kept behind the counter or in locked cases.
c. Pharmacies must maintain a logbook of sales of regulated products.
d. All of the above statements are true.

19. The FDA oversees all but which of the following?

a. Medical devices
b. Medications
c. Vaccines
d. Hazardous waste

20. All but which of the following can be an advantage of a solid dosage form?

a. More accurate dosing
b. Releases medication over a longer period of time
c. Can be used in unconscious patients
d. Longer shelf life than other dosage forms

21. Which of the following is the abbreviation for "before meals"?

a. ac
b. pm
c. pc
d. ad

22. How many grams each of urea 10% cream and 40% cream should be mixed to prepare 30 grams of urea 15% cream?

a. 5 g of urea 10% cream and 25 g of urea 40% cream
b. 18 g of urea 10% cream and 12 g of urea 40% cream
c. 20 g of urea 10% cream and 10 g of urea 40% cream
d. 25 g of urea 10% cream and 5 g of urea 40% cream

23. All but which of the following classes of medications requires a Medication Guide (MedGuide)?

a. Anticonvulsants
b. Thyroid products
c. Antidepressants
d. NSAIDs

24. Which of the following medications is the generic name for Flexeril?

a. Metaxalone
b. Cyclobenzaprine
c. Gabapentin
d. Alendronate

25. **The ISMP is an organization that tracks which of the following?**

    a. Prescription drug costs
    b. Insurance fraud
    c. Medication errors
    d. All of the above

26. **Which of the following is represented by the abbreviation "NS"?**

    a. Nasal solution
    b. No substitution
    c. No salt
    d. Normal saline

27. **All but which of the following medications is a transdermal patch?**

    a. Vivelle-Dot
    b. Abilify
    c. Transderm-Scop
    d. Fentanyl

28. **Patients initiated on sotalol should be monitored in a hospital during the start of therapy to minimize the risk of which of the following side effects?**

    a. Induced arrhythmia
    b. Dehydration
    c. Kidney failure
    d. Hyperglycemia

29. **Which of the following medications is the brand name for ezetimibe?**

    a. Zetia
    b. Crestor
    c. Welchol
    d. Zocor

30. **A drug recall in which there is reasonable probability of serious adverse health consequences or death with the use or exposure of the violative substance is a _____.**

    a. Class I recall
    b. Class II recall
    c. Class III recall
    d. Class IV recall

31. A medication has a wholesale cost of $13.89 and retails for $24.99. The dispensing cost is $3.40. What is the pharmacy's net profit?

   a. $6.30
   b. $7.70
   c. $8.50
   d. $11.10

32. Which of the following are elements of aseptic technique?

   a. Good personal hygiene
   b. Sterile work area
   c. Sterile ingredients
   d. All of the above

33. All but which of the following may issue pharmaceutical recalls?

   a. Wholesaler
   b. FDA
   c. FDA order under statutory authority
   d. Manufacturer

34. Convert 42°Celsius to Fahrenheit.

   a. 83.6°F
   b. 94.3°F
   c. 107.6°F
   d. 109.7°F

35. Which of the following medications is classified as a COX-2 inhibitor?

   a. Diltiazem
   b. Sucralfate
   c. Celecoxib
   d. Warfarin

36. A _____ occurs when an order for a product is billed by the wholesaler but shipped from a different location, such as the manufacturer.

   a. point-of-sale
   b. direct purchase
   c. drop-ship
   d. manufacturer purchase

37. **Which of the following types of container should be used with a medication that requires an airtight seal?**

    a. Polyvinyl chloride (PVC) container
    b. Hermetic container
    c. Amber container
    d. Glass container

38. **St. John's wort is a commonly used natural product for the treatment of which of the following conditions?**

    a. GI distress
    b. Insomnia
    c. Depression
    d. Diabetes

39. **Ampules should not be opened in which of the following directions?**

    a. Towards oneself
    b. Towards the HEPA filter of a laminar flow hood
    c. Towards other sterile products in a laminar flow hood
    d. All of the above

40. **Calculate how many milliliters must be dispensed for the following prescription: Cefdinir 125 mg/5 mL, ½ tsp po bid x 10d**

    a. 25 mL
    b. 50 mL
    c. 60 mL
    d. 75 mL

41. **According to federal law, DEA records must be kept for a minimum of _____ years.**

    a. two
    b. three
    c. four
    d. five

42. **A/an _____ route of administration bypasses the gastrointestinal tract.**

    a. non-parenteral
    b. oral
    c. parenteral
    d. enteral

43. A prescription calls for 500 mL of 0.75% ranitidine solution. How many milliliters of 0.25% ranitidine solution will be needed to prepare the prescription?

    a. 760 mL
    b. 900 mL
    c. 1500 mL
    d. 1800 mL

44. A prescription calls for heparin 1000 units subcutaneously every 12 hours. Multi-dose vials are available that have a concentration of 10,000 units/mL. How many milliliters of heparin should be administered per dose?

    a. 0.1 mL
    b. 0.2 mL
    c. 0.5 mL
    d. 0.7 mL

45. Robitussin AC contains which of the following controlled substances?

    a. Hydrocodone
    b. Codeine
    c. Oxycodone
    d. Morphine

46. Convert the following Roman numeral to an Arabic number: VIII

    a. 2
    b. 8
    c. 13
    d. 18

47. Which of the following medications is used in the treatment of GERD?

    a. Omeprazole
    b. Metformin
    c. Celecoxib
    d. Meloxicam

48. Which of the following laws provides tax and licensing incentives to manufacturers for the development of drugs for the treatment of rare diseases and conditions?

    a. Omnibus Budget Reconciliation Act of 1990
    b. Americans with Disabilities Act of 1990
    c. Orphan Drug Act of 1983
    d. Food, Drug, and Cosmetic Act of 1938

49. Which of the following suffixes refers to blood?

a. -algia
b. -rrhea
c. -uria
d. -emia

50. The use of MAOIs and SSRIs concurrently can cause which of the following potentially fatal conditions?

a. Renal toxicity
b. Rhabdomyolysis
c. Serotonin syndrome
d. Hypotension

51. When compounding emulsions, solutions, and suspensions, the weight of each filled container (corrected for tare weight), should be between which of the following percentages of the labeled volume for each container?

a. 85% and 100%
b. 95% and 100%
c. 95% and 105%
d. 100% and 110%

52. Which of the following medications contains omega-3 fatty acids (EPA and DHA)?

a. TriCor
b. Depakote
c. Lovaza
d. Nexium

53. A maximum of _____ refills can be authorized for a Schedule V controlled substance.

a. one
b. five
c. six
d. ten

54. Magnesium hydroxide can be used to treat which of the following conditions?

a. Allergic rhinitis
b. Fever
c. Constipation
d. Diarrhea

55. All but which of the following is typically found in a patient profile?

a. Third-party provider information
b. Marital status
c. Medications the patient is taking
d. Drug allergies

56. Which of the following medications is classified as an NSAID?

a. Prednisone
b. Meloxicam
c. Clopidogrel
d. Acetaminophen

57. An order is received for 1.5 liters of D5W, to be infused over 24 hours. If the IV administration set is calibrated to deliver 40 gtts/mL, what will the flow rate be in gtts/minute? (round answer to the nearest whole number)

a. 29 gtts/min
b. 33 gtts/min
c. 38 gtts/min
d. 42 gtts/min

58. Which of the following medications is the generic name for Tenormin?

a. Amlodipine
b. Escitalopram
c. Nifedipine
d. Atenolol

59. In which of the following circumstances can a prescription for a Schedule II controlled substance be partially filled?

a. The prescription is for a terminally ill patient.
b. The prescription is for a patient in a hospital.
c. The patient has been on the prescribed medication for at least twelve consecutive months.
d. The prescriber authorizes refills.

60. Which of the following medications is the brand name for alprazolam?

a. Ativan
b. Xanax
c. Levaquin
d. Seroquel

61. Iodine is an element that is important in the production of which of the following substances in the body?

    a. Estrogen
    b. Testosterone
    c. Thyroid hormone
    d. Histamine

62. Which pharmacokinetic phase involves the transport of drugs by the blood to other parts of the body?

    a. Metabolism
    b. Distribution
    c. Excretion
    d. Absorption

63. Mixing liquids and semisoft dosage forms is best done using a _____ mortar and pestle.

    a. Wedgwood
    b. ceramic
    c. porcelain
    d. glass

64. All but which of the following medications should be prepared in a biological safety cabinet?

    a. Etoposide
    b. Doxorubicin
    c. Cisplatin
    d. Vancomycin

65. Convert 20% to a ratio strength.

    a. 1:5
    b. 1:10
    c. 1:20
    d. 1:25

66. HMG-CoA reductase inhibitors are commonly known as which of the following?

    a. Beta-blockers
    b. Proton pump inhibitors
    c. Statins
    d. Diuretics

67. An oral prescription for a Schedule II controlled substance can be issued if all but which of the following criteria are met?

 a. It is an emergency situation.
 b. The drug prescribed and quantity dispensed is enough for the emergency period only.
 c. The prescriber states that the oral prescription is sufficient and a hardcopy prescription will not be sent.
 d. The pharmacist makes a good-faith effort to ensure the identity of the prescriber.

68. Which of the following medications is used to treat a fungal infection?

 a. Ketoconazole
 b. Valacyclovir
 c. Cephalexin
 d. Amoxicillin

69. Which of the following administration routes delivers a medication directly into the bloodstream through a vein?

 a. Subcutaneous
 b. Intramuscular
 c. Intravenous
 d. Enteral

70. Which of the following is another name for vitamin D3?

 a. Calcitonin
 b. Cholecalciferol
 c. Ergocalciferol
 d. Calcidiol

71. Luer-Lok syringes must be used whenever possible for manipulating which of the following types of drugs?

 a. Colored drugs
 b. Hazardous drugs
 c. Acidic drugs
 d. Sterile drugs

72. Which of the following medications is the generic name for Boniva?

 a. Gabapentin
 b. Ibandronate
 c. Fluoxetine
 d. Alendronate

73. Diflucan belongs to which of the following classes of medication?

a. Antiviral
b. Antibiotic
c. Antifungal
d. Antipyretic

74. All but which of the following are required to be on an outpatient prescription label?

a. Directions for use
b. Number of refills permitted
c. Lot number of medication
d. Name of prescriber

75. All but which of the following is true regarding a laminar flow hood?

a. The laminar flow hood should be operated for at least thirty minutes before use.
b. Gloves do not need to be worn when working inside a laminar flow hood.
c. Surfaces should be cleaned with 70% isopropyl alcohol.
d. Manipulations should be performed at least six inches inside the laminar flow hood.

76. Which of the following drugs are composed of both natural and synthetic molecules?

a. Plant-derived drugs
b. Semi-synthetic drugs
c. Synthetic drugs
d. Mineral-derived drugs

77. Which of the following medications is classified as a skeletal muscle relaxant?

a. Metoprolol tartrate
b. Pravastatin
c. Methocarbamol
d. Metformin

78. A pharmacist adds 108 milliliters of acetic acid to water to prepare a total volume of 2 quarts. What is the percentage of acetic acid?

a. 5.7%
b. 6.3%
c. 10.8%
d. 11.4%

79. Which of the following medications is the brand name for fluticasone?

a. Nasacort
b. Flonase
c. Nasonex
d. Astelin

80. Translate the following sig into patient directions: i supp pr q6h prn

a. Insert one suppository vaginally every six hours as needed.
b. Insert one suppository rectally every six hours as needed.
c. Insert one suppository rectally every six hours.
d. Insert one suppository rectally every six hours and at bedtime.

81. Which of the following medications is used to treat migraines?

a. Sumatriptan
b. Pioglitazone
c. Fluvastatin
d. Olanzapine

82. Prescriptions for Schedule III-V controlled substances are valid for _____ from the date written.

a. thirty days
b. sixty days
c. ninety days
d. six months

83. All but which of the following are components of the Isotretinoin Safety and Risk Management Act of 2004?

a. Prescribers, patients, and pharmacies must be enrolled in iPledge.
b. Isotretinoin prescriptions can be filled for a ninety-day supply.
c. All patients must undergo blood tests during treatment.
d. Female patients must undergo monthly pregnancy tests.

84. To reduce contamination while compounding sterile products, gloves should routinely be disinfected with _____.

a. soap
b. 70% isopropyl alcohol
c. bleach
d. ammonia

85. **All but which of the following medications is an H2 receptor antagonist?**

    a. Loratadine
    b. Cimetidine
    c. Famotidine
    d. Ranitidine

86. **Velvachol is an example of which of the following types of ointment base?**

    a. Oleaginous ointment base
    b. Oil-in-water emulsion base
    c. Water-in-oil emulsion base
    d. Absorption ointment base

87. **Convert ½ grain to milligrams.**

    a. 16.2 mg
    b. 32.5 mg
    c. 64.8 mg
    d. 97.2 mg

88. **The maximum weighable quantity that can be measured using a Class III pre-scription balance is _____.**

    a. 100 grams
    b. 110 grams
    c. 120 grams
    d. 130 grams

89. **All but which of the following is true regarding sterile water for injection USP?**

    a. It contains antimicrobial agents.
    b. It can be used for the preparation of parenteral products.
    c. It is water for injection packaged and rendered sterile.
    d. None of the above

90. **A medication that has "01/2018" listed as the expiration date on the manufacturer's container would have an actual expiration date of _____.**

    a. 12/31/2017
    b. 01/01/2018
    c. 01/31/2018
    d. 02/01/2018

91. Which of the following medications is used to treat anxiety?

a. Alprazolam
b. Fluvastatin
c. Metformin
d. Calciprotriene

92. Calculate the days supply for the following prescription: Hycodan 1.5 mg-5 mg/5 mL, 1 tsp q4-6h prn, dispense 120 mL

a. 3 days
b. 4 days
c. 6 days
d. 10 days

93. Which of the following is a set of specific instructions for making a compounded product?

a. Compound formula
b. Master formula
c. Repackaging formula
d. None of the above

94. Which of the following should be considered when selecting a wholesaler?

a. Return policy
b. Delivery rate
c. Pricing
d. All of the above

95. Which of the following natural products is commonly used to treat nausea and motion sickness?

a. Saw palmetto
b. Fish oil
c. Ginger
d. Soy

96. All but which of the following medications should include the auxiliary label "Take on an Empty Stomach"?

a. Fosamax
b. Augmentin
c. Synthroid
d. Boniva

97. The Beers List is a guideline that identifies potentially harmful and inappropriate medications for _____ patients.

a. pediatric
b. elderly
c. pregnant
d. hospitalized

98. Which of the following medications is the brand name for tamsulosin?

a. Avodart
b. Hytrin
c. Rapaflo
d. Flomax

99. Antacids that contain aluminum can cause which of the following side effects?

a. Diarrhea
b. Constipation
c. Bleeding
d. Headache

100. Which of the following medications is used in the treatment of tuberculosis?

a. Isoniazid
b. Doxepin
c. Telmisartan
d. Bumetanide

ANSWER KEY

1. C
Eszopiclone is the generic name for Lunesta.

2. B
$$\frac{1 \text{ cap}}{\text{dose}} \times \frac{4 \text{ doses}}{\text{day}} \times 10 \text{ days} = 40 \text{ capsules}$$

3. B
A closed formulary is comprised of a restricted list of medications selected by a committee, and only certain drugs in each drug class are covered.

4. D
The intravenous route of administration provides the quickest onset.

5. D
The abbreviation "PO" means "by mouth."

6. D
Vibramycin is the brand name for doxycycline hyclate.

7. C
The amount of solvent required to dissolve a particular amount of drug is referred to as solubility.

8. D
A direct purchase occurs when a pharmacy orders a product directly from the manufacturer.

9. C
The sig "i tab po tid x 7d" translates to "Take one tablet by mouth three times a day for seven days."

10. C
Triamterene, eplerenone, and spironolactone are potassium-sparing diuretics.

11. A
A pharmacy that dispenses an investigational new drug is involved with procurement and storage of the drug, monitoring and reporting of adverse drug reactions, and patient education.

12. D
The prefix "peri-" means "surrounding."

13. B
Zolpidem is classified as a hypnotic.

14. C
Personnel hand hygiene and garbing procedures should take place in the ante-area.

15. C
The Pure Food and Drug Act of 1906 prohibits interstate commerce of misbranded and adulterated food and drugs.

16. A
TriCor is the brand name for fenofibrate.

17. B
75 mcg × 1 mg/1000 mcg = 0.075 mg

18. A
The Combat Methamphetamine Epidemic Act of 2005 applies to nonprescription drug products containing ephedrine, pseudoephedrine, and phenylpropanolamine. It states that regulated products must be kept behind the counter or in locked cases, and pharmacies must maintain a logbook of sales of regulated products.

19. D
The FDA oversees medical devices, medications, and vaccines.

20. C
Advantages of a solid dosage form include more accurate dosing, releasing medication over a longer period of time, and longer shelf life than other dosage forms.

21. A
The abbreviation for "before meals" is "ac."

22. D

Percentage		Parts
40%		5 parts
	15%	
10%		25 parts
		30 total parts

Step 1: Quantity of 10% urea cream: 30 g × 25/30 = 25 g
Step 2: Quantity of 40% urea cream: 30 g × 5/30 = 5 g

23. B
Anticonvulsants, antidepressants, and NSAIDs require a Medication Guide (MedGuide).

24. B
Cyclobenzaprine is the generic name for Flexeril.

25. C
The ISMP is an organization that tracks medication errors.

26. D
The abbreviation "NS" means "normal saline."

27. B
Vivelle-Dot, Transderm-Scop, and Fentanyl are transdermal patches.

28. A
Patients initiated on sotalol should be monitored in a hospital during the start of therapy to minimize the risk of induced arrhythmia.

29. A
Zetia is the brand name for ezetimibe.

30. A
A drug recall in which there is a reasonable probability of serious adverse health consequences or death is a Class I recall.

31. B
$24.99 – ($13.89 + 3.40) = $7.70

32. D
Good personal hygiene, a sterile work area, and sterile ingredients are elements of aseptic technique.

33. A
Pharmaceutical recalls may be issued by the manufacturer, the FDA, or by FDA order under statutory authority.

34. C
(42 × 1.8) + 32 = 107.6°F

35. C
Celecoxib is classified as a COX-2 inhibitor.

36. C
A drop-ship occurs when an order for a product is billed by the wholesaler but shipped from a different location, such as the manufacturer.

37. B
A hermetic container should be used with a medication that requires an airtight seal.

38. C
St. John's wort is a commonly used natural product for the treatment of depression.

39. D

Ampules should not be opened towards oneself, towards the HEPA filter of a laminar flow hood, or towards other sterile products in a laminar flow hood.

40. B

$$\frac{2.5 \text{ mL}}{\text{dose}} \times \frac{2 \text{ doses}}{\text{day}} \times 10 \text{ days} = 50 \text{ mL}$$

41. A

According to federal law, DEA records must be kept for a minimum of two years.

42. C

A parenteral route of administration bypasses the gastrointestinal tract.

43. C

Step 1: $0.25\% \times x \text{ mL} = 0.75\% \times 500 \text{ mL}$
Step 2: $0.25x = 375$
Step 3: $x = 1500 \text{ mL}$

44. A

$1000 \text{ units} \times 1 \text{ mL}/10{,}000 \text{ units} = 0.1 \text{ mL}$

45. B

Robitussin AC contains codeine.

46. B

VIII: V + III = 5 + 3 = 8

47. A

Omeprazole is used in the treatment of GERD.

48. C

The Orphan Drug Act of 1983 provides tax and licensing incentives to manufacturers for the development of drugs for the treatment of rare diseases and conditions.

49. D

The suffix "-emia" refers to blood.

50. C

The use of MAOIs and SSRIs concurrently can cause serotonin syndrome.

51. D

When compounding emulsions, solutions, and suspensions, the weight of each filled container (corrected for tare weight), should be between 100% and 110% of the labeled volume for each container.

52. C

Lovaza contains omega-3 fatty acids (EPA and DHA).

53. B
A maximum of five refills can be authorized for a Schedule V controlled substance.

54. C
Magnesium hydroxide can be used to treat constipation.

55. B
Third-party provider information, medications the patient is taking, and drug allergies are typically found in a patient profile.

56. B
Meloxicam is classified as an NSAID.

57. D
$$\frac{1500 \text{ mL}}{1440 \text{ min}} \times \frac{40 \text{ gtts}}{\text{mL}} = 41.7 \text{ gtts/min} = 42 \text{ gtts/min}$$

58. D
Atenolol is the generic name for Tenormin.

59. A
A prescription for a Schedule II controlled substance can be partially filled if it is written for a terminally ill patient.

60. B
Xanax is the brand name for alprazolam.

61. C
Iodine is an element that is important in the production of thyroid hormone in the body.

62. B
Distribution is the pharmacokinetic phase that involves the transport of drugs by the blood to other parts of the body.

63. D
Mixing liquids and semisoft dosage forms is best done using a glass mortar and pestle.

64. D
Etoposide, doxorubicin, and cisplatin should be prepared in a biological safety cabinet.

65. A
Step 1: $\dfrac{20}{100} = \dfrac{1}{x}$

Step 2: $20x = 100$

Step 3: $x = 5$, therefore the ratio is 1:5.

66. C
HMG-CoA reductase inhibitors are commonly known as statins.

67. C
An oral prescription for a Schedule II controlled substance can be issued if it is an emergency situation, the drug prescribed and quantity prescribed are enough for the emergency period only, the prescriber provides a written prescription to the pharmacy within seven days of the oral order, and the pharmacist makes a good-faith effort to ensure the identity of the prescriber.

68. A
Ketoconazole is used to treat a fungal infection.

69. C
The intravenous administration route delivers a medication directly into the bloodstream through a vein.

70. B
Cholecalciferol is another name for vitamin D3.

71. B
Luer-Lok syringes must be used whenever possible for manipulating hazardous drugs.

72. B
Ibandronate is the generic name for Boniva.

73. C
Diflucan belongs to the antifungal class of medications.

74. C
The directions for use, number of refills permitted, and the name of the prescriber are required to be on an outpatient prescription label.

75. B
A laminar flow hood should be operated for at least thirty minutes before use, surfaces should be cleaned with 70% isopropyl alcohol, and manipulations should be performed at least six inches inside the laminar flow hood.

76. B
Semi-synthetic drugs are composed of both natural and synthetic molecules.

77. C
Methocarbamol is classified as a skeletal muscle relaxant.

78. A
Step 1: $\dfrac{108\text{ mL}}{1892\text{ mL}} = \dfrac{x}{100}$

Step 2: $1892x = 10{,}800$

Step 3: $x = 5.7$ mL of acetic acid in 100 mL of solution, therefore the percentage of acetic acid is 5.7%.

79. B
Flonase is the brand name for fluticasone.

80. B
The sig "i supp pr q6h prn" translates to "Insert one suppository rectally every six hours as needed."

81. A
Sumatriptan is used to treat migraines.

82. D
Prescriptions for Schedule III-V controlled substances are valid for six months from the date written.

83. B
The Isotretinoin Safety and Risk Management Act of 2004 requires that prescribers, patients, and pharmacies must be enrolled in iPledge, all patients must undergo blood tests during treatment, and female patients must undergo monthly pregnancy tests.

84. B
To reduce contamination while compounding sterile products, gloves should routinely be disinfected with 70% isopropyl alcohol.

85. A
Cimetidine, famotidine, and ranitidine are H2 receptor antagonists.

86. B
Velvachol is an example of an oil-in-water emulsion base.

87. B
½ gr × 65 mg/gr = 32.5 mg

88. C
The maximum weighable quantity that can be measured using a Class III prescription balance is 120 grams.

89. A
Sterile water for injection USP does not contain antimicrobial agents.

90. C
A medication that has "01/2018" listed as the expiration date on the manufacturer's container would have an actual expiration date of 01/31/2018.

91. A
Alprazolam is used to treat anxiety.

92. B
$$120 \text{ mL} \times \frac{\text{dose}}{5 \text{ mL}} \times \frac{\text{day}}{6 \text{ doses}} = 4 \text{ days supply}$$

93. B
A master formula is a set of specific instructions for making a compounded product.

94. D
The return policy, delivery rate, and pricing should all be considered when selecting a wholesaler.

95. C
Ginger is a natural product commonly used to treat nausea and motion sickness.

96. B
Fosamax, Synthroid, and Boniva should include the auxiliary label "Take on an Empty Stomach."

97. B
The Beers List is a guideline that identifies potentially harmful and inappropriate medications for elderly patients.

98. D
Flomax is the brand name for tamsulosin.

99. B
Antacids that contain aluminum can cause constipation.

100. A
Isoniazid is used in the treatment of tuberculosis.

COMPREHENSIVE EXAM 3

QUESTIONS

1. Which of the following medications is a Schedule II controlled substance?

    a. Nuvigil
    b. Intuniv
    c. Vyvanse
    d. Xanax

2. When the amount of solvent necessary to dissolve a drug is greater than the quantity requested in the prescription, the final preparation will most likely be in which of the following forms?

    a. Syrup
    b. Solution
    c. Emulsion
    d. Suspension

3. The required air quality for an ante-area is typically _____.

    a. ISO Class 1
    b. ISO Class 3
    c. ISO Class 5
    d. ISO Class 8

4. Which of the following describes the meaning of the root word "derm"?

    a. Bone
    b. Skin
    c. Lung
    d. Stomach

5. Which of the following medications is used as a smoking cessation aid?

    a. Benicar
    b. Chantix
    c. Lovaza
    d. Premarin

6. Which of the following may affect the availability of medications?

    a. Unusually high demand
    b. Recalls
    c. Issues with manufacturing
    d. All of the above

7. **Calculate how many milliliters must be dispensed for the following prescription: Amoxicillin 400 mg/5 mL, 1 tsp po q8h x 10d**

a. 75 mL
b. 100 mL
c. 150 mL
d. 180 mL

8. **Which of the following medications decrease levels of oral contraceptives?**

a. Rifampin
b. Furosemide
c. Liothyronine
d. Ketoconazole

9. **Which of the following pieces of personal protective equipment can be reused during a work shift by employees working in a sterile compounding area if it is not visibly soiled?**

a. Gown
b. Gloves
c. Face mask
d. All of the above

10. **All but which of the following are true regarding the Durham-Humphrey Amendment of 1951?**

a. Authorized verbal prescriptions and refills of prescription drugs
b. Established separate categories for prescription and over-the-counter drugs
c. Required that all drugs be labeled with adequate directions for use unless they include the label, "Caution: Federal Law Prohibits Dispensing Without a Prescription."
d. Required that drugs be proven safe and effective

11. **A _____ refers to pharmacies that come together and agree to purchase products from a specific wholesaler, who agrees to provide products to the pharmacies in the group at a reduced cost.**

a. direct vendor group
b. purchasing group
c. discounted purchase group
d. prime vendor group

12. **How many milliliters are in two teaspoons?**

a. 5 mL
b. 7.5 mL
c. 10 mL
d. 15 mL

13. Which of the following medications is classified as an antipsychotic?

a. Phenergan
b. Reglan
c. Zyprexa
d. Avapro

14. All but which of the following is true regarding Medication Guides (MedGuides)?

a. They do not need to be dispensed with refills.
b. They are FDA-approved patient handouts.
c. They are required for certain medications.
d. They can help patients avoid serious adverse events.

15. A TPN order calls for 80 milliequivalents of potassium chloride. Stock vials contain 2 mEq/mL. How many milliliters of potassium chloride should be used?

a. 15 mL
b. 20 mL
c. 30 mL
d. 40 mL

16. Which of the following medications is the generic name for Elavil?

a. Clonazepam
b. Enalapril
c. Amitriptyline
d. Trazodone

17. Which of the following organizations oversees the Vaccine Adverse Event Reporting System?

a. CDC
b. DEA
c. TJC
d. USP

18. Which of the following medications is used to treat opioid dependence?

a. Zyban
b. Suboxone
c. Keppra
d. Actos

19. **How many milliliters should be dispensed for a prescription that calls for one pint?**

    a. 120 mL
    b. 240 mL
    c. 473 mL
    d. 946 mL

20. **Pharmacy technicians must complete the required number of continuing education hours every _____ in order to maintain certification.**

    a. six months
    b. one year
    c. two years
    d. three years

21. **Which of the following is another name for vitamin D2?**

    a. Ergocalciferol
    b. Calcidiol
    c. Cholecalciferol
    d. Calcitonin

22. **Which of the following information is required to be included on an outpatient prescription label?**

    a. Medication lot number
    b. Prescriber's DEA number
    c. Name and address of the pharmacy
    d. All of the above

23. **Convert the following Roman numeral to an Arabic number: VI**

    a. 4
    b. 5
    c. 6
    d. 11

24. **Which of the following types of formularies includes aspects of both open and closed formularies?**

    a. Restricted formulary
    b. Open formulary
    c. Closed formulary
    d. Tiered formulary

25. How many milliliters are in 2.5 teaspoons?

a. 5 mL
b. 7.5 mL
c. 10 mL
d. 12.5 mL

26. Which of the following organizations requires the segregation of medications in order to prevent medication errors and to promote the proper use of medications?

a. OSHA
b. TJC
c. FDA
d. DEA

27. All but which of the following medications is classified as an SSRI?

a. Citalopram
b. Duloxetine
c. Sertraline
d. Paroxetine

28. Translate the following sig into patient directions: i tab po bid x 10d

a. Take one tablet by mouth three times a day for ten days.
b. Take one tablet by mouth once a day for ten days.
c. Take one tablet by mouth twice a day for ten days.
d. Take one tablet by mouth once a day for ten doses.

29. Sharps containers should have all but which of the following qualities?

a. They should be marked with a fill line.
b. They should be leak-proof on the sides and bottom.
c. They should be made of heavy-duty plastic.
d. They should not have a lid.

30. Which of the following medications is used in the treatment of narcolepsy?

a. Wellbutrin
b. Lasix
c. Provigil
d. Desyrel

31. **Which of the following parts of Medicare covers durable medical equipment (DME)?**

    a. Part A
    b. Part B
    c. Part C
    d. Part D

32. **Which of the following DAW codes should be used if no product selection is indicated?**

    a. DAW 0
    b. DAW 1
    c. DAW 2
    d. DAW 3

33. **Which of the following natural products causes enzyme induction and should not be used with certain prescription medications?**

    a. St. John's wort
    b. Cranberry
    c. Peppermint oil
    d. Fish oil

34. **Glucophage is indicated for which of the following conditions?**

    a. Diabetes
    b. Gout
    c. Hypertension
    d. Asthma

35. **How many tablespoons are in 240 milliliters?**

    a. 16 tbsp
    b. 20 tbsp
    c. 24 tbsp
    d. 48 tbsp

36. **Which of the following suffixes refers to flow or discharge?**

    a. -osis
    b. -rrhea
    c. -sclerosis
    d. -uria

37. An ampule requires the use of a _____ needle.

    a. large bore
    b. filter
    c. short
    d. long

38. An auxiliary label indicating "Take with Plenty of Water" should be included with which of the following medications?

    a. Zocor
    b. Norvasc
    c. Bactrim
    d. Januvia

39. Select controlled medications may be sold without a prescription if they belong to which of the following schedules?

    a. Schedule I
    b. Schedule III
    c. Schedule V
    d. All controlled medications must be dispensed pursuant to a prescription.

40. Cephalexin 250-mg capsules cost $69.40/100 capsules. How much will a patient be charged for 30 capsules if the pharmacy adds a 35% markup on cost and a $6.00 dispensing fee?

    a. $20.82
    b. $28.11
    c. $31.27
    d. $34.11

41. When preparing a nonhazardous medication, which of the following syringe sizes should be selected?

    a. The size largest to the volume being measured
    b. The size smallest to the volume being measured
    c. The size closest to the volume being measured
    d. Any size is appropriate

42. All but which of the following abbreviations indicates that a dosage form is extended- or sustained-release?

    a. SR
    b. XL
    c. LA
    d. IR

43. Which of the following medications is the brand name for terbinafine?

a. Lamictal
b. Nizoral
c. Lamisil
d. Voltaren

44. A patient is to receive 1.5 teaspoons of a medication twice daily. How many milliliters per day will the patient receive?

a. 10 mL/day
b. 15 mL/day
c. 18 mL/day
d. 30 mL/day

45. All but which of the following medications is used to prevent blood clots?

a. Plavix
b. Coumadin
c. Celebrex
d. Xarelto

46. Which of the following laws defines and regulates dietary supplements?

a. Pure Food and Drug Act of 1906
b. Food and Drug Administration Safe Medical Devices Act of 1990
c. Dietary Supplement Health and Education Act of 1994
d. Food, Drug, and Cosmetic Act of 1938

47. A prescriber's DEA number would be required on a prescription for which of the following medications?

a. Adderall
b. Zocor
c. Wellbutrin
d. Cialis

48. Which of the following medications is classified as a benzodiazepine?

a. Prednisone
b. Naproxen
c. Cimetidine
d. Lorazepam

49. **A prescriber orders a 1 liter bag of IV fluids to be administered at a flow rate of 100 mL/hr. How many hours will the bag last?**

    a. 8 hours
    b. 10 hours
    c. 12 hours
    d. 16 hours

50. **Which of the following medications is classified as an opioid?**

    a. Meperidine
    b. Carisoprodol
    c. Meloxicam
    d. Cyclobenzaprine

51. **Which of the following medications is used to treat hyperthyroidism?**

    a. Propylthiouracil
    b. Levothyroxine
    c. Armour Thyroid
    d. Liothyronine

52. **All interior working surfaces of a laminar flow hood should be cleaned with which of the following products prior to use?**

    a. Detergent crystals
    b. Tap water
    c. 70% isopropyl alcohol
    d. Alkaline detergent

53. **All but which of the following is typically the first letter of a prescriber's DEA number?**

    a. A
    b. B
    c. F
    d. Y

54. **Which of the following administration routes delivers a medication through the skin or mucous membrane?**

    a. Epidural
    b. Topical
    c. Subcutaneous
    d. Intravenous

55. The beyond-use date for a low-risk compounded sterile product stored at room temperature cannot exceed _____.

    a. 24 hours
    b. 48 hours
    c. 72 hours
    d. 96 hours

56. Convert 0.05% to a ratio strength.

    a. 1:50
    b. 1:100
    c. 1:200
    d. 1:2000

57. Which of the following references contains drug pricing information such as the average wholesale price (AWP) and suggested retail price?

    a. Red Book
    b. The Merck Index
    c. American Drug Index
    d. United States Pharmacopeia

58. Ophthalmic solutions are used to administer medication to which of the following areas of the body?

    a. Nails
    b. Eyes
    c. Lungs
    d. Rectum

59. Which of the following is the abbreviation for "twice a day"?

    a. qid
    b. bid
    c. tid
    d. tiw

60. Which of the following medications is the generic name for Pravachol?

    a. Atenolol
    b. Ibandronate
    c. Pravastatin
    d. Amitriptyline

61. A prescription for a Schedule II controlled substance that is being partially filled for a terminally ill or long-term care facility patient is valid for _____ from the date of issue.

   a. ten days
   b. thirty days
   c. sixty days
   d. ninety days

62. Which of the following medications is the generic name for Nexium?

   a. Omeprazole
   b. Prednisone
   c. Fluticasone
   d. Esomeprazole

63. If 250 milliliters of D50W is infused, how many grams of dextrose will the patient receive?

   a. 1.25 g
   b. 125 g
   c. 250 g
   d. 500 g

64. When measuring a liquid, the substance should not constitute less than _____ of the graduate's capacity.

   a. 5%
   b. 10%
   c. 15%
   d. 20%

65. All but which of the following is an example of a Schedule I controlled substance?

   a. Heroin
   b. Ecstasy
   c. Opium
   d. Cocaine

66. Which of the following is the proper injection method for insulin?

   a. Intramuscular
   b. Subcutaneous
   c. Intrathecal
   d. None of the above

67. Which of the following medications is classified as an alpha-blocker?

a. Tamsulosin
b. Sotalol
c. Amlodipine
d. Propranolol

68. Which of the following concentrations of sodium chloride is isotonic with body cells?

a. 0.009% NaCl
b. 0.09% NaCl
c. 0.9% NaCl
d. 9% NaCl

69. Translate the following sig into patient directions: i tab SL prn chest pain

a. Take one tablet as needed for chest pain.
b. Place one tablet under the tongue as needed for chest pain.
c. Take one tablet after meals as needed for chest pain.
d. Place one tablet under the tongue at bedtime as needed for chest pain.

70. Which of the following medications is the generic name for Tamiflu?

a. Famciclovir
b. Telmisartan
c. Oseltamivir
d. Amantadine

71. A prescription calls for cefdinir 250 mg/5 mL with a dose of two teaspoons twice daily. How many milligrams will the patient receive in each dose?

a. 250 mg
b. 375 mg
c. 500 mg
d. 700 mg

72. Which of the following laws encourages the creation of both generic and name brand drugs by streamlining the approval process and extending patent life?

a. Prescription Drug Marketing Act of 1987
b. Drug Price Competition and Patent Restoration Act of 1984
c. Durham-Humphrey Amendment of 1951
d. Food, Drug, and Cosmetic Act of 1938

73. Patients should remain upright for at least thirty minutes after taking which of the following medications?

    a. Alendronate
    b. Raloxifene
    c. Estradiol
    d. Clomiphene

74. USP <795> addresses which of the following topics regarding the compounding of non-sterile products?

    a. Beyond-use dating
    b. Ingredient selection
    c. Quality control
    d. All of the above

75. Which of the following medications is classified as a corticosteroid?

    a. Rabepazole
    b. Donepezil
    c. Bisoprolol
    d. Prednisone

76. Which of the following ointment bases is the most occlusive?

    a. Oleaginous ointment base
    b. Water-in-oil emulsion base
    c. Oil-in-water emulsion base
    d. Water-miscible ointment base

77. Which organ in the body is primarily responsible for the metabolism of drugs?

    a. Brain
    b. Liver
    c. Kidney
    d. Spleen

78. Which of the following medications is considered a long-acting insulin?

    a. Insulin lispro (Humalog)
    b. Insulin glargine (Lantus)
    c. Insulin aspart (Novolog)
    d. Regular insulin (Humulin)

79. All but which of the following is true regarding weights used for a Class III prescription balance?

a. The weights can be touched by hand.
b. The weights cannot be dropped or dented.
c. The weights must be clean when stored.
d. All of the above are correct.

80. It is important to avoid fermented foods when taking which of the following classes of medication?

a. Proton pump inhibitors
b. Diuretics
c. Antibiotics
d. MAOIs

81. Which of the following dosage forms are concentrated aqueous preparations of a sugar or sugar substitute?

a. Elixir
b. Syrup
c. Tincture
d. Suspension

82. Which of the following medications is classified as an anticoagulant?

a. Aspirin
b. Clopidogrel
c. Warfarin
d. Dipyridamole

83. Calculate how many drops per day a patient will use for the following prescription: Combigan, i gtt ou bid

a. 2 gtts/day
b. 4 gtts/day
c. 8 gtts/day
d. 10 gtts/day

84. All but which of the following information is required to be included on the label for unit-dose medications?

a. Name of drug
b. Pharmacist's initials
c. Lot number of medication
d. Beyond-use date

85. All but which of the following medications is classified as an ACE inhibitor?

a. Vasotec
b. Prinivil
c. Lotensin
d. Zyloprim

86. Which of the following is true regarding expiration dates?

a. They are assigned by the pharmacy.
b. If the expiration date reads "04/2020," the product actually expires 04/01/2020.
c. They are assigned by the manufacturer.
d. They can be assigned by the wholesaler.

87. Which of the following medications is used to treat an arrhythmia?

a. Enalapril
b. Digoxin
c. Montelukast
d. Ranitidine

88. During a controlled substance inventory, which of the following classes of medication can have their total quantity estimated?

a. Schedule II medications
b. Schedule III, IV, and V medications in package sizes less than or equal to 1000
c. Schedule III, IV, and V medications in package sizes greater than 1000
d. All of the above

89. Which of the following terms refers to the colorings, flavorings, and preservatives found in drug products?

a. Inert ingredients
b. Active ingredients
c. Essential ingredients
d. Extra ingredients

90. Which of the following types of inventory ordering occurs when an item is deducted from the inventory as it is dispensed and is automatically reordered?

a. Just-in-time ordering
b. Purchase ordering
c. Point-of-sale ordering
d. Direct sale ordering

91. Black cohosh and evening primrose oil are natural products commonly used to treat symptoms associated with which of the following conditions?

a. Dementia
b. Menopause
c. Nausea
d. Depression

92. Which of the following is represented by the abbreviation "D5W"?

a. 5 mg dextrose in water
b. 5% dextrose in water
c. 50 g dextrose in water
d. 50% dextrose in water

93. Which of the following pharmacokinetic phases involves chemical processes that change drug molecules?

a. Metabolism
b. Absorption
c. Excretion
d. Distribution

94. Which of the following over-the-counter medications can increase the risk of heart attack and stroke?

a. Antihistamines
b. Antacids
c. NSAIDs
d. Probiotics

95. Which of the following describes the proper administration for medications that are to be taken buccally?

a. They should be placed under the tongue.
b. They should be injected subcutaneously.
c. They should be swallowed.
d. They should be placed between the gums and cheek.

96. Which of the following medications is used to treat nausea?

a. Promethazine
b. Allopurinol
c. Sitagliptin
d. Carvedilol

97. Calculate how many milliliters must be dispensed for the following prescription: Prednisolone 15 mg/5 mL, 1.5 tsp po qd x 7d

a. 35 mL
b. 40.5 mL
c. 52.5 mL
d. 60 mL

98. All but which of the following vitamins are fat soluble?

a. Vitamin A
b. Vitamin B6
c. Vitamin D
d. Vitamin K

99. Which of the following can be described as the study of what the body does to a drug?

a. Therapeutics
b. Pharmacokinetics
c. Pharmaceutics
d. Pharmacodynamics

100. Which of the following antibiotics is safe to use in patients with a severe allergy to penicillin?

a. Azithromycin
b. Amoxicillin
c. Cephalexin
d. Cefuroxime

ANSWER KEY

1. C
Vyvanse is a Schedule II controlled substance.

2. D
When the amount of solvent necessary to dissolve a drug is greater than the quantity requested in the prescription, the final preparation will most likely be a suspension.

3. D
The required air quality for an ante-area is typically ISO Class 8.

4. B
The meaning of the root word "derm" is "skin."

5. B
Chantix is used as a smoking cessation aid.

6. D
Unusually high demand, recalls, and issues with manufacturing may affect the availability of medications.

7. C
$$\frac{5 \text{ mL}}{\text{dose}} \times \frac{3 \text{ doses}}{\text{day}} \times 10 \text{ days} = 150 \text{ mL}$$

8. A
Rifampin decreases levels of oral contraceptives.

9. A
A gown can be reused during a work shift by employees working in a sterile compounding area if it is not visibly soiled.

10. D
The Durham-Humphrey Amendment of 1951 authorized verbal prescriptions and refills of prescription drugs, established separate categories for prescription and over-the-counter drugs, and required that all drugs be labeled with adequate directions for use unless they include the label, "Caution: Federal Law Prohibits Dispensing Without a Prescription."

11. B
A purchasing group refers to pharmacies that come together and agree to purchase products from a specific wholesaler, who agrees to provide products to the pharmacies in the group at a reduced cost.

12. C
2 tsp × 5 mL/tsp = 10 mL

13. C
Zyprexa is classified as an antipsychotic.

14. A
Medication Guides (MedGuides) are FDA-approved patient handouts that are required for certain medications each time they are filled. They can help patients avoid serious adverse events.

15. D
80 mEq × 1 mL/2 mEq = 40 mL

16. C
Amitriptyline is the generic name for Elavil.

17. A
The CDC and the FDA oversee the Vaccine Adverse Event Reporting System.

18. B
Suboxone is used to treat opioid dependence.

19. C
473 milliliters should be dispensed for a prescription that calls for one pint.

20. C
Pharmacy technicians must complete the required number of continuing education hours every two years in order to maintain certification.

21. A
Ergocalciferol is another name for vitamin D2.

22. C
The name and address of the pharmacy is required to be included on an outpatient prescription label.

23. C
VI: V + I = 5 + 1 = 6

24. A
A restricted formulary includes aspects of both open and closed formularies.

25. D
2.5 tsp x 5 mL/tsp = 12.5 mL

26. B
The Joint Commission requires the segregation of medications in order to prevent medication errors and to promote the proper use of medications.

27. B
Citalopram, sertraline and paroxetine are classified as SSRIs.

28. C
The sig "i tab po bid x 10d" translates to "Take one tablet by mouth twice a day for ten days."

29. D
Sharps containers should be marked with a fill line, leak-proof on the sides and bottom, and have a lid. They should be made of heavy-duty plastic.

30. C
Provigil is used in the treatment of narcolepsy.

31. B
Medicare Part B covers durable medical equipment.

32. A
DAW 0 should be used if no product selection is indicated.

33. A
St. John's wort is a natural product that causes enzyme induction and should not be used with certain prescription medications.

34. A
Glucophage is indicated for diabetes.

35. A
240 mL × 1 tbsp/15 mL = 16 tbsp

36. B
The suffix "-rrhea" refers to flow or discharge.

37. B
An ampule requires the use of a filter needle.

38. C
An auxiliary label indicating "Take with Plenty of Water" should be included with Bactrim.

39. C
Select controlled medications may be sold without a prescription if they belong to Schedule V.

40. D
Step 1: $69.40 ÷ 100 capsules = 0.694 per capsule × 30 capsules = $20.82
Step 2: $20.82 + (20.82 × 35%) = 28.107 + $6.00 = 34.107 = $34.11

41. C
When preparing a nonhazardous medication, the syringe size closest to the volume being measured should be selected.

42. D
SR, XL, and LA are abbreviations that indicate a dosage form is extended- or sustained-release.

43. C
Lamisil is the brand name for terbinafine.

44. B
$$\frac{1.5 \text{ tsp}}{\text{dose}} \times \frac{2 \text{ doses}}{\text{day}} \times \frac{5 \text{ mL}}{\text{tsp}} = 15 \text{ mL/day}$$

45. C
Plavix, Coumadin, and Xarelto are used to prevent blood clots.

46. C
The Dietary Supplement Health and Education Act of 1994 defines and regulates dietary supplements.

47. A
A prescriber's DEA number would be required on a prescription for Adderall.

48. D
Lorazepam is classified as a benzodiazepine.

49. B
1000 mL × 1 hr/100 mL = 10 hours

50. A
Meperidine is classified as an opioid.

51. A
Propylthiouracil is used to treat hyperthyroidism.

52. C
All interior working surfaces of a laminar flow hood should be cleaned with 70% isopropyl alcohol prior to use.

53. D
A, B, or F are typically the first letters of a prescriber's DEA number.

54. B
The topical administration route delivers a medication through the skin or mucous membrane.

55. B
The beyond-use date for a low-risk compounded sterile product stored at room temperature cannot exceed 48 hours.

56. D

Step 1: $\dfrac{0.05}{100} = \dfrac{1}{x}$

Step 2: $0.05x = 100$

Step 3: $x = 2000$, therefore the ratio is 1:2000.

57. A

The *Red Book* contains drug pricing information such as the average wholesale price (AWP) and suggested retail price.

58. B

Ophthalmic solutions are used to administer medication to the eyes.

59. B

The abbreviation for "twice a day" is "bid."

60. C

Pravastatin is the generic name for Pravachol.

61. C

A prescription for a Schedule II controlled substance that is being partially filled for a terminally ill or long-term care facility patient is valid for sixty days from the date of issue.

62. D

Esomeprazole is the generic name for Nexium.

63. B

Step 1: $\dfrac{50\text{ g}}{100\text{ mL}} = \dfrac{x\text{ g}}{250\text{ mL}}$

Step 2: $100x = 12{,}500$

Step 3: $x = 125$ g

64. D

When measuring a liquid, the substance should not constitute less than 20% of the graduate's capacity.

65. D

Heroin, ecstasy, and opium are examples of a Schedule I controlled substance.

66. B

Subcutaneous administration is the proper injection method for insulin.

67. A

Tamsulosin is classified as an alpha-blocker.

68. C

0.9% NaCl is isotonic with body cells.

69. B
The sig "i tab SL prn chest pain" translates to "Place one tablet under the tongue as needed for chest pain."

70. C
Oseltamivir is the generic name for Tamiflu.

71. C
$$\frac{10 \text{ mL}}{\text{dose}} \times \frac{250 \text{ mg}}{5 \text{ mL}} = 500 \text{ mg/dose}$$

72. B
The Drug Price Competition and Patent Restoration Act of 1984 encourages the creation of both generic and name brand drugs by streamlining the approval process and extending patent life.

73. A
Patients should remain upright for at least thirty minutes after taking alendronate.

74. D
Among several other areas, USP <795> addresses beyond-use dating, ingredient selection, and quality control for the compounding of non-sterile products.

75. D
Prednisone is classified as a corticosteroid.

76. A
Oleaginous ointment bases are the most occlusive of the choices provided.

77. B
The liver is primarily responsible for the metabolism of drugs.

78. B
Insulin glargine (Lantus) is considered a long-acting insulin.

79. A
The weights used for a Class III prescription balance should never be touched by hand, cannot be dropped or dented, and must be clean when stored.

80. D
It is important to avoid fermented foods when taking MAOIs.

81. B
A syrup is a concentrated aqueous preparation of a sugar or sugar substitute.

82. C
Warfarin is classified as an anticoagulant.

83. B
$$\frac{2 \text{ gtts}}{\text{dose}} \times \frac{2 \text{ doses}}{\text{day}} = 4 \text{ gtts/day}$$

84. B
The name of the drug, lot number of the medication, and beyond-use date are required to be included on the label for unit-dose medications.

85. D
Vasotec, Prinivil, and Lotensin are classified as ACE inhibitors.

86. C
Expiration dates are assigned by the manufacturer.

87. B
Digoxin is used to treat an arrhythmia.

88. B
During a controlled substance inventory, Schedule III, IV, and V medications in package sizes less than or equal to 1000 can have their total quantity estimated.

89. A
Inert ingredients refer to the colorings, flavorings, and preservatives found in drug products.

90. C
Point-of-sale ordering occurs when an item is deducted from the inventory as it is dispensed and is automatically reordered.

91. B
Black cohosh and evening primrose oil are natural products commonly used to treat symptoms associated with menopause.

92. B
The abbreviation "D5W" means "5% dextrose in water."

93. A
Metabolism is the pharmacokinetic phase that involves chemical processes that change drug molecules.

94. C
NSAIDs can increase the risk of heart attack and stroke.

95. D
Medications that are to be taken buccally should be placed between the gums and cheek.

96. A
Promethazine is used to treat nausea.

97. C
$$\frac{7.5 \text{ mL}}{\text{dose}} \times \frac{1 \text{ dose}}{\text{day}} \times 7 \text{ days} = 52.5 \text{ mL}$$

98. B

Vitamin A, vitamin D, and vitamin K are fat soluble.

99. B

Pharmacokinetics can be described as the study of what the body does to a drug.

100. A

Azithromycin is safe to use in patients with a severe allergy to penicillin.

COMPREHENSIVE EXAM 4

COMPREHENSIVE EXAM

QUESTIONS

1. Which of the following is a Schedule I controlled substance?

    a. OxyContin
    b. Heroin
    c. Ritalin
    d. Halcion

2. Cetirizine belongs to which of the following pharmacologic categories?

    a. Analgesic
    b. Decongestant
    c. Antihistamine
    d. Expectorant

3. Which of the following laws requires that manufacturers provide proof of drug effectiveness and safety?

    a. Pure Food and Drug Act of 1906
    b. Food, Drug, and Cosmetic Act of 1938
    c. Durham-Humphrey Amendment of 1951
    d. Kefauver-Harris Amendment of 1962

4. Which of the following is the abbreviation for "at bedtime"?

    a. pm
    b. hs
    c. ac
    d. noc

5. Which of the following medications is the generic name for Zantac?

    a. Esomeprazole
    b. Loratadine
    c. Ranitidine
    d. Metoprolol

6. When the amount of solvent necessary to dissolve a drug is less than the quantity requested in the prescription, the final preparation will most likely be in which of the following forms?

    a. Suspension
    b. Solution
    c. Oil-in-water emulsion
    d. Water-in-oil emulsion

7. **Which of the following medications is a short-acting bronchodilator that can be used as a rescue inhaler?**

    a. Advair
    b. Symbicort
    c. Dulera
    d. ProAir

8. **Which of the following tablet dosage forms is designed to be dissolved in liquid before administration?**

    a. Buccal
    b. Effervescent
    c. Sublingual
    d. Enteric-coated

9. **The required air quality for a buffer area is _____.**

    a. ISO Class 1
    b. ISO Class 5
    c. ISO Class 7
    d. ISO Class 8

10. **Which of the following is true regarding medications with a high turnover rate?**

    a. The medications are rarely used.
    b. The medications should be kept at minimum stock levels.
    c. They should be ordered regularly in appropriate quantities to ensure there is enough stock to fill prescriptions.
    d. None of the above are true.

11. **Translate the following sig into patient directions: i–ii tabs po q4h prn pain**

    a. Take one to two tablets by mouth up to four times a day as needed for pain.
    b. Take one to two tablets by mouth four times a day as needed for pain.
    c. Take one to two tablets by mouth every four hours as needed for pain.
    d. Take one to two tablets by mouth every four hours after meals for pain.

12. **A TPN order calls for 40 milliequivalents of potassium sulfate. Stock vials contain 6 mEq/mL. How many milliliters of potassium sulfate should be used?**

    a. 4.8 mL
    b. 6.7 mL
    c. 9.3 mL
    d. 12.2 mL

13. A biennial inventory of _____ must be conducted according to the Controlled Substances Act.

    a. all prescription medications
    b. controlled substances
    c. chemotherapy medications
    d. All of the above

14. Tall man lettering is an error-prevention strategy used to reduce the risk of which of the following medication errors?

    a. Confusing look-alike and sound-alike drug names
    b. Incorrect dosing
    c. Incorrect directions
    d. Inappropriate medication administration

15. Which of the following is represented by the second letter of a DEA number?

    a. The letter is chosen at random by the DEA.
    b. It is the first letter of the state the prescriber practices in.
    c. It is the first letter of the prescriber's last name at the time of registration with the DEA.
    d. The letter is chosen at random by the prescriber.

16. The suffix "-sclerosis" refers to which of the following conditions?

    a. Tumor
    b. Inflammation
    c. Hardening
    d. Pain

17. How often should the air quality of a laminar flow hood be certified?

    a. Every year
    b. When it is moved to a different location
    c. Anytime it is cleaned
    d. All of the above

18. A patient that is allergic to penicillin may also be allergic to what other class of medications?

    a. Statins
    b. Beta-blockers
    c. Cephalosporins
    d. Sulfonamides

19. **A prescriber orders 250 mg of ciprofloxacin to be taken twice a day for 3 days. How many total grams of ciprofloxacin are prescribed?**

    a. 0.5 g
    b. 1.5 g
    c. 2 g
    d. 3 g

20. **Which of the following patient handouts contains FDA-approved information about important adverse events that can occur with the use of certain medications?**

    a. Package inserts
    b. Medication information leaflet
    c. Medication Guides (MedGuides)
    d. Consumer leaflet

21. **Which of the following medications is classified as an antihyperlipidemic?**

    a. Cimetidine
    b. Pravastatin
    c. Levofloxacin
    d. Glipizide

22. **The reconstitution and transfer of a sterile vial of an antibiotic into one sterile diluent IV bag is an example of _____ compounding.**

    a. low-risk
    b. medium-risk
    c. high-risk
    d. transfer

23. **Which of the following over-the-counter medications is used for the treatment of cold sores?**

    a. Zicam
    b. Abreva
    c. Chloraseptic
    d. Benadryl

24. **Which of the following copies of DEA Form 222 is sent to the supplier after it is filled out by the pharmacy?**

    a. Copy 1
    b. Copy 2
    c. Copy 3
    d. Copies 1 and 2

25. Quinolone antibiotics should not be administered concurrently with which of the following?

    a. Analgesics
    b. Antihistamines
    c. Dairy products
    d. All of the above

26. A "May Cause Discoloration of the Urine" auxiliary label would be appropriate for which of the following medications?

    a. Pravastatin
    b. Metoprolol tartrate
    c. Phenazopyridine
    d. Amoxicillin

27. All but which of the following medications require refrigeration for storage prior to dispensing?

    a. Insulin
    b. Pred Forte
    c. NuvaRing
    d. Xalatan

28. Which of the following types of compounding equipment should not be swabbed with 70% isopropyl alcohol prior to use for a sterile preparation?

    a. A needle shaft
    b. Rubber stopper of a vial
    c. Neck of an ampule
    d. All of the above should be swabbed with 70% isopropyl alcohol.

29. Which of the following is an example of an extended-release dosage form that can be split?

    a. Effexor XR
    b. Wellbutrin XL
    c. Toprol-XL
    d. Cardizem SR

30. Which of the following medications is classified as an antihistamine?

    a. Motrin
    b. Tylenol
    c. NasalCrom
    d. Allegra

31. Calculate how many grams of Cerave are needed for the following prescription:

Menthol crystals	
Camphor crystals	aa 0.5%
Salicylic acid powder	2%
Cerave	qs 30 g

   a. 27.2 g
   b. 28.3 g
   c. 29.1 g
   d. 30.2 g

32. Prescriptions written for a Schedule III-V controlled substance may be partially filled how many times?

   a. Zero
   b. Once
   c. Twice
   d. None of the above

33. Used needles and sharps should be disposed of in a _____.

   a. recycling bin
   b. sharps container
   c. trash can
   d. trash bag

34. All but which of the following medications is classified as an ARB?

   a. Prozac
   b. Diovan
   c. Cozaar
   d. Avapro

35. Convert 6 fluid ounces to milliliters.

   a. 90 mL
   b. 110 mL
   c. 180 mL
   d. 200 mL

36. Which of the following medications is the brand name for latanoprost?

   a. Travatan Z
   b. Durezol
   c. Lumigan
   d. Xalatan

37. According to USP <797>, pharmacy personnel who compound high-risk level sterile products must have their aseptic technique evaluated _____.

    a. monthly
    b. quarterly
    c. twice a year
    d. annually

38. Which of the following pharmacokinetic phases involves the removal of a drug from the body?

    a. Distribution
    b. Excretion
    c. Absorption
    d. Metabolism

39. Which of the following describes the proper administration for sublingual dosage forms?

    a. They should be injected subcutaneously.
    b. They should be swallowed.
    c. They should be placed under the tongue.
    d. They should be placed between the gums and cheek.

40. Which of the following medications is the generic name for ProAir?

    a. Tiotropium
    b. Fluticasone
    c. Salmeterol
    d. Albuterol

41. A one gram vial of an antibiotic states that 7.8 milliliters of sterile water should be added to the dry powder to produce a solution containing 100 mg/mL. What is the powder volume of the vial?

    a. 1.8 mL
    b. 2.2 mL
    c. 2.7 mL
    d. 3.1 mL

42. Which of the following antitussive medications contains codeine?

    a. Mucinex DM
    b. Delsym
    c. Robitussin AC
    d. None of the above

43. To ensure fluid transfer into an IV bag, a needle that is greater than _____ should be used to pierce the injection port.

    a. 1/16-inches
    b. 3/16-inches
    c. 1/8-inches
    d. 3/8-inches

44. Which of the following describes how many digits are in each segment of an NDC number?

    a. 2, 4, 5
    b. 3, 5, 2
    c. 5, 4, 2
    d. 6, 2, 3

45. Calculate how many capsules are needed to fill the following prescription: Fluoxetine 20 mg, 3 caps po qam, dispense 90 day supply

    a. 30 capsules
    b. 90 capsules
    c. 180 capsules
    d. 270 capsules

46. Which of the following references provides the most comprehensive compounding information?

    a. American Drug Index
    b. Remington: The Science and Practice of Pharmacy
    c. Orange Book
    d. United States Pharmacopeia

47. All but which of the following items are considered durable medical equipment (DME)?

    a. Syringes
    b. Crutches
    c. Walker
    d. Cane

48. Calculate how many drops per day a patient will use for the following prescription: Ciprofloxacin 0.3%, 2 gtts od qid

    a. 2 gtts/day
    b. 4 gtts/day
    c. 8 gtts/day
    d. 10 gtts/day

49. All but which of the following medications is a Schedule II controlled substance?

a. Ritalin
b. Fiorinal
c. Percocet
d. Adderall

50. All but which of the following medications are sensitive to light?

a. Nitroprusside
b. Furosemide
c. Iron
d. Calcium

51. Translate the following sig into patient directions: 1 tsp po q4h prn cough

a. Take one tablespoonful by mouth every four hours as needed for cough.
b. Take one teaspoonful by mouth every four hours as needed for cough.
c. Take one teaspoonful by mouth four times a day as needed for cough.
d. Take one tablespoonful by mouth four times a day as needed for cough.

52. When preparing a hazardous medication, the measured volume should not exceed _____ capacity of the syringe.

a. 25%
b. 50%
c. 75%
d. 85%

53. All but which of the following is an example of a Schedule III or IV controlled substance?

a. Alprazolam
b. Zolpidem
c. Oxycodone
d. Zaleplon

54. Which of the following medications is indicated for seizure prevention?

a. Lansoprazole
b. Naproxen
c. Eszopiclone
d. Valproic acid

55. One quart of a solution contains 30 grams of an active ingredient. Calculate the w/v%.

    a. 2.9%
    b. 3.2%
    c. 5.7%
    d. 6.3%

56. USP <797> addresses which of the following areas regarding the compounding of sterile products?

    a. Microbial contamination risk levels
    b. Employee use of aseptic technique
    c. Environmental monitoring
    d. All of the above

57. Otic solutions are used to administer medication to which of the following areas of the body?

    a. Eyes
    b. Ears
    c. Skin
    d. Mouth

58. Which of the following DEA forms is used to report the theft of controlled substances?

    a. Form 41
    b. Form 106
    c. Form 222
    d. Form 224

59. Convert 1:1000 to a percent strength.

    a. 0.001%
    b. 0.01%
    c. 0.1%
    d. 1%

60. Which of the following natural products is associated with liver toxicity?

    a. Cinnamon
    b. Kava kava
    c. Zinc
    d. Soy

61. A reaction in which the actions of a drug are inhibited or decreased by the actions of another drug is a/an _____ interaction.

   a. synergistic
   b. antagonistic
   c. summation
   d. protagonist

62. A maximum of _____ refills can be authorized for a Schedule III controlled substance prescription.

   a. zero
   b. one
   c. three
   d. five

63. Which of the following laws allowed for the creation of the prescription drug benefit for Medicare beneficiaries known as Medicare Part D?

   a. Medicare Prescription Drug, Improvement, and Modernization Act of 2003
   b. Omnibus Budget and Reconciliation Act of 1990
   c. Health Insurance Portability and Accountability Act of 1996
   d. Resource Conservation and Recovery Act

64. Which of the following describes the proper administration for lozenge dosage forms?

   a. They should be swallowed immediately.
   b. They should be slowly dissolved in the mouth.
   c. They should be dissolved in liquid.
   d. They should be applied to the skin.

65. A patient is to receive 1.5 grams of cefazolin every 8 hours. The pharmacy has a 20 milliliter vial that has a concentration of 1000 mg/5 mL. How many milliliters are needed per dose?

   a. 5 mL
   b. 7.5 mL
   c. 12 mL
   d. 25 mL

66. Which of the following medications is the generic name for Levemir?

   a. Insulin glargine
   b. Insulin aspart
   c. Insulin lispro
   d. Insulin detemir

67. Which of the following dosage forms is a sweetened, hydroalcoholic solution?

   a. Syrup
   b. Suspension
   c. Liniment
   d. Elixir

68. Which of the following medications is the brand name for temazepam?

   a. Ambien
   b. Xanax
   c. Restoril
   d. Provigil

69. A 500 milliliter bag of 0.45% NS is to be infused over six hours. If the calibration of the IV tubing is 10 gtts/mL, how many drops per minute will there be? (round answer to the nearest whole number)

   a. 12 gtts/min
   b. 14 gtts/min
   c. 18 gtts/min
   d. 20 gtts/min

70. Which of the following laws permits prescriptions to be called into a pharmacy over the telephone?

   a. Durham-Humphrey Act of 1951
   b. Kefauver-Harris Amendment of 1962
   c. Food, Drug, and Cosmetic Act of 1938
   d. Omnibus Budget Reconciliation Act of 1990

71. Which of the following DAW codes should be selected if the prescriber indicates that a generic substitution is permitted, but the generic product is temporarily unavailable so the brand product is dispensed instead?

   a. DAW 1
   b. DAW 2
   c. DAW 3
   d. DAW 8

72. Which of the following medications is used in the treatment of dementia?

   a. Xalatan
   b. Aricept
   c. Pamelor
   d. Buspar

73. The beyond-use date for a medium-risk compounded sterile product stored at room temperature cannot exceed _____.

a. ten hours
b. twenty hours
c. thirty hours
d. forty hours

74. Which of the following statements is false regarding the use of graduates to measure liquids?

a. Conical graduates are more accurate for measuring liquids than cylindrical graduates.
b. The correct reading is at the bottom of the meniscus.
c. The reading must be done at eye level.
d. A graduate with a capacity equal to or slightly larger than the volume to be measured should be selected.

75. Which of the following describes the meaning of the root word "pulmo"?

a. Skin
b. Lung
c. Stomach
d. Heart

76. How many milliliters are in 2 tablespoons?

a. 5 mL
b. 15 mL
c. 20 mL
d. 30 mL

77. Which of the following medications is used in the treatment of gout?

a. Zithromax
b. Neurontin
c. Desyrel
d. Zyloprim

78. Which of the following ointment bases is suitable to use for drugs that are hydrolyzed by water?

a. Water-in-oil emulsion base
b. Oil-in-water emulsion base
c. Absorption ointment base
d. Oleaginous ointment base

79. **Medications that require refrigeration for storage should generally be kept within which temperature range?**

    a. 0° and 5°C (32° and 41°F)
    b. 2° and 8°C (36° and 46°F)
    c. 8° and 12°C (46° and 54°F)
    d. 15° and 20°C (59° and 68°F)

80. **Which of the following types of intravenous administration is a one-time, rapid injection of medication into the bloodstream?**

    a. IV push
    b. IV infusion
    c. IV line
    d. IV drip

81. **Which of the following medications is classified as an opioid analgesic?**

    a. Flexeril
    b. Soma
    c. OxyContin
    d. Neurontin

82. **Which of the following is assigned by a manufacturer and used to identify a specific batch of medication?**

    a. Expiration date
    b. NDC number
    c. Lot number
    d. Product code

83. **Which of the following describes the proper disposal method for cytotoxic medications?**

    a. Return to the wholesaler
    b. Destroy with biohazardous waste items
    c. Return to the manufacturer
    d. Contact the EPA

84. **Women who are pregnant or planning to become pregnant should take which of the following supplements to prevent neural tube defects?**

    a. Iron
    b. Vitamin D
    c. Folic acid
    d. Calcium

85. A maximum of _____ refills can be authorized for Percocet.

    a. zero
    b. one
    c. three
    d. five

86. When billing a third-party provider, which of the following relationship holder codes is usually selected for a patient that is a child of the primary cardholder?

    a. 00
    b. 01
    c. 02
    d. 03

87. Which of the following describes how often a Medication Guide (MedGuide) should be given to a patient that is taking a medication that requires receipt of one?

    a. Annually
    b. Each time the prescription is filled
    c. Every six months
    d. The first time the prescription is filled

88. Hyzaar is a combination of which of the following medications?

    a. Hydrochlorothiazide and losartan
    b. Amlodipine and benazepril
    c. Hydrochlorothiazide and triamterene
    d. Sitagliptin and metformin

89. All but which of the following is an example of an electrolyte that may be in a TPN solution?

    a. Sodium chloride
    b. Potassium acetate
    c. Calcium gluconate
    d. Insulin

90. Which of the following is represented by the abbreviation "D5NS"?

    a. 0.5% dextrose in normal saline
    b. 5 mg dextrose in normal saline
    c. 5% dextrose in normal saline
    d. 50 g dextrose in normal saline

91. Which of the following medications is the generic name for Omnicef?

a. Cefdinir
b. Ciprofloxacin
c. Cephalexin
d. Cefazolin

92. Which of the following medications is used in the treatment of epilepsy?

a. Keppra
b. Vesicare
c. Levsin
d. Dyazide

93. Calculate how many capsules are needed to fill the following prescription: Cephalexin 250 mg, i cap po q6h x 7d

a. 21
b. 28
c. 35
d. 42

94. Which of the following prefixes means painful or difficult?

a. Ante-
b. Dys-
c. Hemi-
d. Peri-

95. According to USP <795>, the beyond-use date for compounded water-containing formulations is _____ when stored under refrigeration in the absence of other data.

a. 14 days
b. 30 days
c. 60 days
d. 90 days

96. Which of the following is a common side effect of Augmentin?

a. Dry cough
b. Photosensitivity
c. GI upset
d. Insomnia

97. Which of the following can affect the absorption of a medication?

a. Route of administration
b. Patient weight
c. Patient age
d. All of the above

98. Which of the following medications is classified as an SSRI?

a. Prozac
b. Fosamax
c. Effexor
d. Altace

99. All but which of the following are examples of a solid dosage form?

a. Suppository
b. Tablet
c. Capsule
d. Ointment

100. Which of the following medications is used to treat hypertension?

a. Paroxetine
b. Diphenhydramine
c. Glyburide
d. Lisinopril

ANSWER KEY

1. B
Heroin is a Schedule I controlled substance.

2. C
Cetirizine is an antihistamine.

3. D
The Kefauver-Harris Amendment of 1962 requires that manufacturers provide proof of drug effectiveness and safety.

4. B
The abbreviation for "at bedtime" is "hs."

5. C
Ranitidine is the generic name for Zantac.

6. B
When the amount of solvent necessary to dissolve a drug is less than the quantity requested in the prescription, the final preparation will most likely be a solution.

7. D
ProAir is a short-acting bronchodilator that can be used as a rescue inhaler.

8. B
Effervescent tablets are designed to be dissolved in liquid before administration.

9. C
The required air quality for a buffer area is ISO Class 7.

10. C
Medications with a high turnover rate should be ordered regularly in appropriate quantities to ensure there is enough stock to fill prescriptions.

11. C
The sig "i–ii tabs po q4h prn pain" translates to "Take one to two tablets by mouth every four hours as needed for pain."

12. B
40 mEq × 1 mL/6 mEq = 6.7 mL

13. B
A biennial inventory of controlled substances must be conducted according to the Controlled Substances Act.

14. A
Tall man lettering is an error-prevention strategy used to reduce the risk of confusing look-alike and sound-alike drug names.

15. C
The second letter of a DEA number represents the first letter of the prescriber's last name at the time of registration with the DEA.

16. C
The suffix "-sclerosis" refers to hardening.

17. B
The air quality of a laminar flow hood should be certified every six months, when it is moved to a different location, or if damage is suspected.

18. C
A patient that is allergic to penicillin may also be allergic to cephalosporins.

19. B
$$\frac{0.25 \text{ g}}{\text{dose}} \times \frac{2 \text{ doses}}{\text{day}} \times 3 \text{ days} = 1.5 \text{ g}$$

20. C
Medication Guides (MedGuides) are patient handouts that contain FDA-approved information about important adverse events that can occur with the use of certain medications.

21. B
Pravastatin is classified as an antihyperlipidemic.

22. A
The reconstitution and transfer of a sterile vial of an antibiotic into one sterile diluent IV bag is an example of low-risk compounding.

23. B
Abreva is an over-the-counter medication used for the treatment of cold sores.

24. D
Copies 1 and 2 of DEA Form 222 are sent to the supplier after they are filled out by the pharmacy.

25. C
Quinolone antibiotics should not be administered concurrently with dairy products.

26. C
A "May Cause Discoloration of the Urine" auxiliary label would be appropriate for phenazopyridine.

27. B
Insulin, NuvaRing, and Xalatan require refrigeration for storage prior to dispensing.

28. A
Needle shafts should never be swabbed with 70% isopropyl alcohol or touched prior to use for a sterile preparation.

29. C
Toprol-XL is an example of an extended-release dosage form that can be split.

30. D
Allegra is classified as an antihistamine.

31. C
Step 1: Menthol crystals: 0.005×30 g $= 0.15$ g
Step 2: Camphor crystals: 0.005×30 g $= 0.15$ g
Step 3: Salicylic acid powder: 0.02×30 g $= 0.6$ g
Step 4: Cerave: 30 g $- (0.15$ g $+ 0.15$ g $+ 0.6$ g$) = 29.1$ g

32. D
Prescriptions written for a Schedule III-V controlled substance may be partially filled an unlimited number of times as long as the total quantity dispensed in all partial fillings does not exceed the total quantity prescribed and all fillings are dispensed within six months of the date of issuance.

33. B
Used needles and sharps should be disposed of in a sharps container.

34. A
Diovan, Cozaar, and Avapro are classified as ARBs.

35. C
6 oz $\times$ 30 mL/oz $= 180$ mL

36. D
Xalatan is the brand name for latanoprost.

37. C
According to USP <797>, pharmacy personnel who compound high-risk level sterile products must have their aseptic technique evaluated twice a year.

38. B
Excretion is the pharmacokinetic phase that involves the removal of a drug from the body.

39. C
Proper administration for sublingual dosage forms is to place them under the tongue.

40. D
Albuterol is the generic name for ProAir.

41. B

Step 1: $\dfrac{100\ mg}{mL} = \dfrac{1000\ mg}{x}$

Step 2: $100x = 1000$

Step 3: $x = 10\ mL$

Step 4: $10\ mL - 7.8\ mL = 2.2\ mL$

42. C

Robitussin AC is an antitussive medication that contains codeine.

43. D

To ensure fluid transfer into an IV bag, a needle that is greater than 3/8-inches should be used to pierce the injection port.

44. C

Each segment of an NDC number has 5, 4, and 2 digits.

45. D

90 days × 3 caps/day = 270 capsules

46. B

Remington: The Science and Practice of Pharmacy provides the most comprehensive compounding information.

47. A

Crutches, a walker, and a cane are considered durable medical equipment.

48. C

$\dfrac{2\ gtts}{dose} \times \dfrac{4\ doses}{day} = 8\ gtts/day$

49. B

Ritalin, Percocet, and Adderall are Schedule II controlled substances.

50. D

Nitroprusside, furosemide, and iron are medications that are sensitive to light.

51. B

The sig "1 tsp po q4h prn cough" translates to "Take one teaspoonful by mouth every four hours as needed for cough."

52. C

When preparing a hazardous medication, the measured volume should not exceed 75% of the capacity of the syringe.

53. C

Alprazolam, zolpidem, and zaleplon are examples of a Schedule III or IV controlled substance.

54. D
Valproic acid is indicated for seizure prevention.

55. B
Step 1: $\dfrac{30 \text{ g}}{946 \text{ mL}} = \dfrac{x \text{ mL}}{100}$

Step 2: $946x = 3000$

Step 3: $x = 3.2$ g of active ingredient in 100 mL of solution, therefore the percentage strength is 3.2%.

56. D
Among several other areas, USP <797> addresses microbial contamination risk levels, employee use of aseptic technique, and environmental monitoring.

57. B
Otic solutions are used to administer medication to the ears.

58. B
DEA Form 106 is used to report the theft of controlled substances.

59. C
Step 1: $\dfrac{1}{1000} = \dfrac{x}{100}$

Step 2: $1000x = 100$

Step 3: $x = 0.1$, therefore the percent strength is 0.1%.

60. B
Kava kava is a natural product associated with liver toxicity.

61. B
A reaction in which the actions of a drug are inhibited or decreased by the actions of another drug is an antagonistic drug interaction.

62. D
A maximum of five refills can be authorized for a Schedule III controlled substance prescription.

63. A
The Medicare Prescription Drug, Improvement, and Modernization Act of 2003 allowed for the creation of the prescription drug benefit for Medicare beneficiaries known as Medicare Part D.

64. B
The proper administration of lozenge dosage forms is to slowly dissolve them in the mouth.

65. B
1.5 g × 5 mL/g = 7.5 mL

66. D
Insulin detemir is the generic name for Levemir.

67. D
An elixir is a sweetened, hydroalcoholic solution.

68. C
The brand name for temazepam is Restoril.

69. B
$$\frac{500 \text{ mL}}{6 \text{ hr}} \times \frac{\text{hr}}{60 \text{ min}} \times \frac{10 \text{ gtts}}{\text{mL}} = 13.9 \text{ gtts/min} = 14 \text{ gtts/min}$$

70. A
The Durham-Humphrey Act of 1951 permits prescriptions to be called into a pharmacy over the telephone.

71. D
DAW 8 should be selected if the prescriber indicates that a generic substitution is permitted, but the generic product is temporarily unavailable so the brand product is dispensed instead.

72. B
Aricept is used in the treatment of dementia.

73. C
The beyond-use date for a medium-risk compounded sterile product stored at room temperature cannot exceed thirty hours.

74. A
Conical graduates are less accurate for measuring liquids than cylindrical graduates.

75. B
The meaning of the root word "pulmo" is "lung."

76. D
2 tbsp × 15 mL/tbsp = 30 mL

77. D
Zyloprim is used in the treatment of gout.

78. D
Oleaginous ointment bases are suitable to use for drugs that are hydrolyzed by water.

79. B
Medications that require refrigeration for storage should generally be kept within 2° and 8°C (36° and 46°F).

80. A
An IV push is a one-time, rapid injection of medication into the bloodstream.

81. C
OxyContin is classified as an opioid analgesic.

82. C
A lot number is assigned by a manufacturer and used to identify a specific batch of medication.

83. B
The proper disposal method for cytotoxic medications is to destroy them with biohazardous waste items.

84. C
Women who are pregnant or planning to become pregnant should take folic acid to prevent neural tube defects.

85. A
A maximum of zero refills can be authorized for Percocet.

86. D
When billing a third-party provider, relationship holder code "03" is usually selected for a patient that is a child of the primary cardholder.

87. B
A Medication Guide (MedGuide) should be given each time a prescription is filled to a patient who is taking a medication that requires receipt of one.

88. A
Hyzaar is a combination of hydrochlorothiazide and losartan.

89. D
Sodium chloride, potassium acetate, and calcium gluconate are examples of an electrolyte that may be in a TPN solution.

90. C
The abbreviation "D5NS" means "5% dextrose in normal saline."

91. A
The generic name for Omnicef is cefdinir.

92. A
Keppra is used in the treatment of epilepsy.

93. B
$$\frac{1 \text{ cap}}{\text{dose}} \times \frac{4 \text{ doses}}{\text{day}} \times 7 \text{ days} = 28 \text{ capsules}$$

94. B
The prefix "dys-" means "painful or difficult."

95. A
According to USP <795>, the beyond-use date for compounded water-containing formulations is 14 days when stored under refrigeration in the absence of other data.

96. C
GI upset is a common side effect of Augmentin.

97. D
The route of administration, the patient's weight, and the patient's age can affect the absorption of a medication.

98. A
Prozac is classified as an SSRI.

99. D
Suppositories, tablets, and capsules are examples of solid dosage forms.

100. D
Lisinopril is used to treat hypertension.

COMPREHENSIVE EXAM 5

QUESTIONS

1. Which of the following supplements is commonly used as a sleep aid?

   a. Acai
   b. Cranberry
   c. Melatonin
   d. Milk thistle

2. Which of the following types of intravenous administration is a slow delivery of medication into a vein over a set period of time?

   a. IV push
   b. IV bolus
   c. IV line
   d. IV infusion

3. Which of the following medications is the generic name for Toprol-XL?

   a. Zolpidem
   b. Pantoprazole
   c. Metoprolol succinate
   d. Metoprolol tartrate

4. Which of the following medications is the brand name for cetirizine?

   a. Benadryl
   b. Allegra
   c. Zyrtec
   d. Claritin

5. Which of the following describes how PAR (periodic automatic replacement) levels of seasonal medications should be adjusted at the end of the season to avoid overstock?

   a. PAR levels should be increased.
   b. PAR levels should be decreased.
   c. PAR levels should be kept the same.
   d. None of the above

6. Lithium is indicated for the treatment of which of the following conditions?

   a. Congestive heart failure
   b. Anxiety
   c. Bipolar disorder
   d. Insomnia

7. Which of the following describes the meaning of the root word "lipo"?

a. Fat
b. Lung
c. Skin
d. Stomach

8. Convert the following Roman numeral to an Arabic number: XII

a. 8
b. 12
c. 17
d. 22

9. The Kefauver-Harris Amendment of 1962 requires that manufacturers do all but which of the following?

a. Supply evidence of drug effectiveness
b. Follow Good Manufacturing Practices set by the government
c. Supply evidence of drug safety
d. Provide adequate directions for use on all drug labels

10. Convert 4 grains to grams.

a. 0.26 g
b. 0.74 g
c. 165.5 g
d. 260 g

11. Which of the following medications is the generic name for Abilify?

a. Ziprasidone
b. Valacyclovir
c. Aripiprazole
d. Escitalopram

12. Which of the following describes the meaning of the prefix "tachy-"?

a. With
b. Out
c. Fast
d. Change

13. All but which of the following medications is used to treat fungal infections?

a. Ketoconazole
b. Clotrimazole
c. Nystatin
d. Amoxicillin

14. Which of the following is true regarding liquid dosage forms?

a. Faster absorption than solid dosage forms
b. Do not usually require special storage
c. Longer shelf life than solid dosage forms
d. None of the above

15. When working in a vertical laminar flow hood, nothing should pass _____ a sterile object.

a. behind
b. in front of
c. above
d. below

16. Which of the following questions regarding a prescription is a pharmacy technician permitted to answer?

a. Potential side effects of the medication
b. Drug interactions that can occur
c. Storage requirements of the medication
d. Name of medication

17. A TPN order calls for 70 milliequivalents of calcium gluconate. Stock vials contain 5 mEq/mL. How many milliliters of calcium gluconate should be used?

a. 10 mL
b. 12 mL
c. 14 mL
d. 16 mL

18. A "Do Not Drink Alcohol" auxiliary label would be appropriate for which of the following medications?

a. Metronidazole
b. Sertraline
c. Azithromycin
d. Hydrochlorothiazide

19. Which of the following medications is the brand name for pantoprazole?

a. Prilosec
b. Protonix
c. Synthroid
d. Lipitor

20. Which of the following medications require a patient package insert?

a. Statins
b. Diuretics
c. Oral contraceptives
d. Antibiotics

21. Which of the following is true regarding the proper storage of frozen medications?

a. Stand-alone freezers should be used.
b. The temperature of the freezer should be monitored monthly.
c. Frozen medications should be stored below 40°F (4°C).
d. All of the above are true.

22. Which of the following medications is used for the treatment of head lice?

a. Ketoconazole
b. Permethrin
c. Hydrocortisone
d. Ciclopirox

23. Which of the following copies of DEA Form 222 must be sent from the supplier to the DEA for drug-tracking purposes?

a. Copy 1
b. Copy 2
c. Copy 3
d. None of the above

24. The reconstitution and transfer of a sterile vial of an antibiotic into one sterile diluent IV bag using a non-sterile syringe would be assigned which of the following risk levels?

a. Low-Risk
b. Medium-Risk
c. High-Risk
d. None of the above

25. Cranberry is commonly used as a supplement for the prevention of which of the following conditions?

a. Urinary tract infection
b. Constipation
c. Kidney stones
d. Rhinitis

26. What is the infusion rate in mL/hour of a 0.5 liter bag of normal saline that is to be infused over 8 hours?

a. 43.5 mL/hr
b. 50.5 mL/hr
c. 62.5 mL/hr
d. 70.5 mL/hr

27. Which of the following is an FDA database for post-marketing drug safety and marketing?

a. FAERS
b. VAERS
c. MedMARx
d. NCCMERP

28. Convert 1700 milliliters to liters.

a. 0.17 L
b. 1.7 L
c. 17 L
d. 170 L

29. Translate the following sig into patient directions: 1000 units IM q week

a. Inject 1000 units under the skin every week.
b. Inject 1000 units immediately and in one week.
c. Inject 1000 units into a muscle every other week.
d. Inject 1000 units into a muscle every week.

30. A pharmacy must register with the DEA to dispense controlled substances by completing which of the following DEA forms?

a. Form 41
b. Form 106
c. Form 222
d. Form 224

31. How many grams each of fluocinonide 0.1% ointment and white petrolatum should be mixed to prepare 120 grams of fluocinonide 0.075% ointment?

   a. 75 g of fluocinonide 0.1% ointment and 45 g of white petrolatum
   b. 80 g of fluocinonide 0.1% ointment and 40 g of white petrolatum
   c. 90 g of fluocinonide 0.1% ointment and 30 g of white petrolatum
   d. 100 g of fluocinonide 0.1% ointment and 20 g of white petrolatum

32. Which of the following needle gauges has the smallest diameter?

   a. 13 gauge
   b. 16 gauge
   c. 20 gauge
   d. 27 gauge

33. Which of the following medications is classified as a fluoroquinolone?

   a. Zithromax
   b. Levaquin
   c. Keflex
   d. Omnicef

34. A child weighing 24.2 pounds is to receive cefdinir 14 mg/kg/day for 10 days. How many milligrams of cefdinir will the child receive per day?

   a. 128 mg/day
   b. 154 mg/day
   c. 227 mg/day
   d. 339 mg/day

35. The Combat Methamphetamine Epidemic Act of 2005 limits the daily and monthly sales of pseudoephedrine-containing products to which of the following quantities?

   a. 1.6 grams/day, 3 grams/month
   b. 2.6 grams/day, 6 grams/month
   c. 3.6 grams/day, 9 grams/month
   d. 4.6 grams/day, 12 grams/month

36. Which of the following concentrations of sodium chloride is hypertonic to body cells?

   a. 0.009% NaCl
   b. 0.09% NaCl
   c. 0.9% NaCl
   d. 9% NaCl

37. Which of the following medications is used to relieve pain caused by a urinary tract infection?

a. Indomethacin
b. Phenazopyridine
c. Bumetanide
d. Acebutolol

38. Convert 240 milliliters to ounces.

a. 4 oz
b. 8 oz
c. 12 oz
d. 16 oz

39. Which of the following dosage forms enters the body through the stomach and intestines?

a. Parenteral
b. Enteral
c. Transdermal
d. Sublingual

40. Xalatan can be stored at room temperature for _____ after it is opened.

a. six weeks
b. eight weeks
c. ten weeks
d. twelve weeks

41. Which of the following medications is the brand name for tiotropium?

a. Spiriva
b. Advair
c. Proventil
d. Flovent

42. Calculate how many total drops a patient will use for the following prescription: Ciprodex 4 gtts au bid x 7d

a. 56 gtts
b. 73 gtts
c. 98 gtts
d. 112 gtts

43. All but which of the following medications is classified as a beta-blocker?

a. Metoprolol
b. Tramadol
c. Carvedilol
d. Propranolol

44. If a pharmacy partially fills a Schedule II controlled substance prescription due to inadequate stock, the pharmacy has _____ to furnish the rest of the medication to the patient.

a. 24 hours
b. 48 hours
c. 72 hours
d. 96 hours

45. Which of the following vitamins is required for calcium absorption?

a. Vitamin A
b. Vitamin D
c. Vitamin E
d. Vitamin K

46. All but which of the following medications is a rapid-acting insulin?

a. Humalog
b. Novolog
c. Apidra
d. Lantus

47. Convert 25% to a ratio strength.

a. 1:2
b. 1:4
c. 1:8
d. 1:12

48. Which of the following medical conditions does a patient have if his/her profile lists the abbreviation "GERD"?

a. Gastroesophageal reflux disease
b. Gastrointestinal bleeding
c. Generalized anxiety disorder
d. Gestational diabetes

49. Which of the following medications is the generic name for Bactroban?

a. Ketoconazole
b. Tretinoin
c. Calcipotriene
d. Mupirocin

50. All but which of the following are true regarding the application of transdermal patches?

a. They should be applied to clean skin.
b. They can be applied to broken skin.
c. They should be applied to skin with minimal hair present.
d. They should be applied to skin that is free of powders, oils, and lotions.

51. Which of the following sets standards concerning the requirements for sterile preparation facilities?

a. USP <797>
b. OSHA
c. ISMP
d. All of the above

52. Which of the following medications is classified as an ACE inhibitor?

a. Paxil
b. Zestril
c. Trileptal
d. Pulmicort

53. Unopened insulin should be stored _____.

a. in a freezer
b. at room temperature
c. in a refrigerator
d. in a refrigerator or freezer

54. Which of the following medications is the generic name for Advair?

a. Salmeterol
b. Ipratropium-albuterol
c. Tiotropium
d. Fluticasone-salmeterol

55. Which of the following is the proper injection method for Lovenox?

  a. Intramuscular
  b. Intradermal
  c. Subcutaneous
  d. None of the above

56. Vitamin K plays a major role in which of the following bodily functions?

  a. Blood clotting
  b. Immunity
  c. Digestion
  d. Calcium absorption

57. A reaction in which the actions of a drug are increased by the actions of another drug is a/an _____ drug interaction.

  a. naturalistic
  b. antagonistic
  c. synergistic
  d. catalytic

58. A pharmacy registration with the DEA must be renewed _____.

  a. every year
  b. every two years
  c. every three years
  d. every five years

59. How many milligrams of a drug are in 120 grams of a 15% cream?

  a. 18 mg
  b. 4500 mg
  c. 8000 mg
  d. 18,000 mg

60. Which of the following dosage forms can be used vaginally or rectally?

  a. Elixir
  b. Enteral
  c. Suppository
  d. Solution

61. A drug product that consists of a filthy, putrid, or decomposed substance would be in violation of which of the following federal laws?

a. Pure Food and Drug Act of 1906
b. Food, Drug, and Cosmetic Act of 1938
c. Durham-Humphrey Act of 1951
d. Kefauver-Harris Amendment of 1962

62. Which of the following medications is the generic name for Neurontin?

a. Pregabalin
b. Nortriptyline
c. Niacin
d. Gabapentin

63. How many milliliters of 25% acetic acid stock solution are required to make 2 ounces of 15% acetic acid solution?

a. 9 mL
b. 18 mL
c. 36 mL
d. 100 mL

64. Patients on warfarin may have an increased bleeding risk if they are also taking all but which of the following medications?

a. Aspirin
b. NSAIDs
c. Antiplatelets
d. Antihistamines

65. All but which of the following are general principles for proper operation of a laminar flow hood?

a. A laminar flow hood should operate only while compounding.
b. A laminar flow hood should be tested and certified every six months, whenever it is moved, or if the filter is damaged.
c. Jewelry and artificial nails should not be worn in a laminar flow hood.
d. Nothing should touch the HEPA filter.

66. Which of the following are considered dietary supplements by the FDA?

a. Vitamins
b. Herbs
c. Amino acids
d. All of the above

67. A "Store in Refrigerator" auxiliary label should be used with which of the following medications?

    a. Morphine liquid
    b. Augmentin suspension
    c. Carafate suspension
    d. Furosemide solution

68. All but which of the following over-the-counter medications is an NSAID?

    a. Tylenol
    b. Aleve
    c. Motrin
    d. Advil

69. Which of the following is represented by the abbreviation "gtt"?

    a. Ointment
    b. Milligram
    c. Drop
    d. Gram

70. Which of the following medications is used for the treatment of nasal congestion?

    a. Sudafed
    b. Maalox
    c. Advil
    d. Prilosec

71. The maximum number of refills permitted for a Schedule II controlled substance prescription is _____.

    a. zero
    b. one
    c. two
    d. five

72. Which of the following dosage forms is an example of a dispersion?

    a. Syrup
    b. Tincture
    c. Suspension
    d. Elixir

73. **Which of the following medications is the brand name for prednisone?**

    a. Medrol
    b. Deltasone
    c. Robaxin
    d. Cozaar

74. **Investigational New Drug Applications are reviewed by which of the following federal agencies?**

    a. DEA
    b. FDA
    c. OSHA
    d. USP

75. **A pharmacy technician can perform all but which of the following duties?**

    a. Update a patient profile
    b. Recommend an over-the-counter medication
    c. Manage medication inventory
    d. Bill a third-party provider

76. **Which of the following types of injections is administered into the top layer of skin?**

    a. Intraperitoneal
    b. Subcutaneous
    c. Intrathecal
    d. Intradermal

77. **Which of the following dosage forms contains the most amount of water?**

    a. Ointments
    b. Lotions
    c. Creams
    d. None of the above contains water.

78. **All but which of the following medications is classified as a calcium channel blocker?**

    a. Tenormin
    b. Norvasc
    c. Cardizem
    d. Verelan

79. **Drug products that are considered to be therapeutically equivalent to other products will have a rating code that begins with which of the following letters?**

    a. A
    b. B
    c. E
    d. X

80. **Which of the following medications is used to treat nausea and vomiting?**

    a. Digoxin
    b. Clonazepam
    c. Ondansetron
    d. Gemfibrozil

81. **Which of the following describes how subcutaneous dosage forms should be administered?**

    a. Applied topically
    b. Injected under the skin
    c. Injected into a vein
    d. Injected into a muscle

82. **All but which of the following medications requires a new prescription for each fill?**

    a. Strattera
    b. Adderall
    c. Vicodin
    d. OxyContin

83. **Which of the following is required when compounding sterile products?**

    a. Air quality testing
    b. Product sterility testing
    c. Use of aseptic technique
    d. All of the above

84. **Which of the following is the correct classification of furosemide?**

    a. Thiazide diuretic
    b. Loop diuretic
    c. Calcium channel blocker
    d. ACE inhibitor

85. **Translate the following sig into patient directions: i cap po qod**

    a. Take one capsule by mouth every day.
    b. Take one capsule by mouth twice a day.
    c. Take one capsule by mouth every other day.
    d. Take one capsule by mouth every week.

86. **In a hospital, which of the following areas consists of patient-specific medication?**

    a. Crash carts
    b. Unit-dose carts
    c. Automated dispensing systems
    d. Floor stock

87. **All but which of the following information is required to be included on an out-patient prescription label?**

    a. Number of refills authorized
    b. Prescriber's NPI number
    c. Name of the drug manufacturer
    d. Name and address of the pharmacy

88. **Which of the following medications is the brand name for oxycodone-acetaminophen?**

    a. Percocet
    b. Vicodin
    c. Tylenol No. 3
    d. Fioricet

89. **Medications that are required to be frozen when stored should generally be kept within which of the following temperature ranges?**

    a. -25° and -10°C (-13° and 14°F)
    b. -10° and -5°C (14° and 23°F)
    c. -5° and 0°C (23° and 32°F)
    d. -5° and 5°C (23° and 41°F)

90. **Which of the following natural products may help lower cholesterol levels?**

    a. Chamomile tea
    b. Echinacea
    c. Red yeast rice
    d. Melatonin

91. Which of the following is true regarding a medication's expiration date?

    a. It is assigned by the wholesaler.
    b. It is assigned by the pharmacy.
    c. It is assigned by the manufacturer.
    d. None of the above are true.

92. Hazardous waste is regulated by which of the following?

    a. Pure Food and Drug Act of 1906
    b. Kefauver-Harris Amendment of 1962
    c. Resource Conservation and Recovery Act
    d. Food, Drug, and Cosmetic Act of 1938

93. Vicodin belongs to which of the following DEA schedules?

    a. Schedule II
    b. Schedule III
    c. Schedule IV
    d. Schedule V

94. Which of the following diabetes medications is classified as a biguanide?

    a. Actos
    b. Glucotrol
    c. Glucophage
    d. Januvia

95. An "Avoid Prolonged Exposure to Sunlight" auxiliary label should be used with which of the following medications?

    a. Isotretinoin
    b. Pravastatin
    c. Montelukast
    d. All of the above

96. Calculate how many capsules are needed to fill the following prescription: Benzonatate 100 mg, ii caps po q8h x 10d

    a. 30
    b. 60
    c. 80
    d. 100

97. Which of the following medications is the brand name for oxybutynin?

a. Detrol LA
b. Ditropan XL
c. Vesicare
d. Levsin

98. All but which of the following medications is available over the counter?

a. Flonase
b. Advair
c. Nasacort
d. Zyrtec

99. The beyond-use date for a high-risk compounded sterile product stored at room temperature cannot exceed _____.

a. 24 hours
b. 48 hours
c. 72 hours
d. 96 hours

100. Heparin can be administered by which of the following routes?

a. Intravenous route
b. Oral route
c. Intramuscular route
d. Intradermal route

ANSWER KEY

1. C
Melatonin is commonly used as a sleep aid.

2. D
An IV infusion is a slow delivery of medication into a vein over a set period of time.

3. C
Metoprolol succinate is the generic name for Toprol-XL.

4. C
Zyrtec is the brand name for cetirizine.

5. B
PAR (periodic automatic replacement) levels of seasonal medications should be decreased at the end of the season to avoid overstock.

6. C
Lithium is indicated for the treatment of bipolar disorder.

7. A
The meaning of the root word "lipo" is "fat."

8. B
XII: 10 + 2 = 12

9. D
The Kefauver-Harris Amendment of 1962 requires that manufacturers supply evidence of drug effectiveness, follow Good Manufacturing Practices set by the government, and supply evidence of drug safety.

10. A
4 gr × 65 mg/gr = 260 mg ÷ 1000 = 0.26 g

11. C
Aripiprazole is the generic name for Abilify.

12. C
The prefix "tachy-" means "fast."

13. D
Ketoconazole, clotrimazole, and nystatin are used to treat fungal infections.

14. A
Liquid dosage forms have faster absorption than solid dosage forms.

15. C
When working in a vertical laminar flow hood, nothing should pass above a sterile object.

16. D
A pharmacy technician is permitted to answer a question regarding the name of a medication.

17. C
70 mEq × 1 mL/5 mEq = 14 mL

18. A
A "Do Not Drink Alcohol" auxiliary label would be appropriate for metronidazole.

19. B
Protonix is the brand name for pantoprazole.

20. C
Oral contraceptives require a patient package insert.

21. A
Stand-alone freezers should be used to store frozen medications.

22. B
Permethrin is used for the treatment of head lice.

23. B
Copy 2 of DEA Form 222 must be sent from the supplier to the DEA for drug-tracking purposes.

24. C
The reconstitution and transfer of a sterile vial of an antibiotic into one sterile diluent IV bag using a non-sterile syringe would be assigned a high-risk level.

25. A
Cranberry is commonly used as a supplement for the prevention of urinary tract infections.

26. C
500 mL/8 hr = 62.5 mL/hr

27. A
FAERS (FDA Adverse Event Reporting Systems) is an FDA database for post-marketing drug safety and marketing.

28. B
1700 mL × 1 L/1000 mL = 1.7 L

29. D
The sig "1000 units IM q week" translates to "Inject 1000 units into a muscle every week."

30. D
A pharmacy must register with the DEA to dispense controlled substances by completing DEA Form 224.

31. C

Percentage		Parts
0.1%		0.075 parts
	0.075%	
0%		0.025 parts
		0.1 total parts

Step 1: Quantity of 0.1% fluocinonide ointment: 120 g × 0.075/0.1 = 90 g
Step 2: Quantity of white petrolatum: 120 g × 0.025/0.1 = 30 g

32. D
A 27 gauge needle has the smallest diameter of the sizes listed.

33. B
Levaquin is classified as a fluoroquinolone.

34. B
Step 1: 24.2 lb × 1 kg/2.2 lb = 11 kg
Step 2: 14 mg/kg/day × 11 kg = 154 mg/day

35. C
The Combat Methamphetamine Epidemic Act of 2005 limits the daily and monthly sales of pseudoephedrine-containing products to 3.6 grams/day and 9 grams/month.

36. D
9% NaCl is hypertonic to body cells.

37. B
Phenazopyridine is used to relieve pain caused by a urinary tract infection.

38. B
240 mL × 1 oz/30 mL = 8 oz

39. B
Enteral dosage forms enter the body through the stomach and intestines.

40. A
Xalatan can be stored at room temperature for six weeks after it is opened.

41. B
Spiriva is the brand name for tiotropium.

42. D

$$\frac{8 \text{ gtts}}{\text{dose}} \times \frac{2 \text{ doses}}{\text{day}} \times 7 \text{ days} = 112 \text{ gtts}$$

43. B

Metoprolol, carvedilol, and propranolol are classified as beta-blockers.

44. C

If a pharmacy partially fills a Schedule II controlled substance prescription due to inadequate stock, the pharmacy has 72 hours to furnish the rest of the medication to the patient.

45. B

Vitamin D is required for calcium absorption.

46. D

Humalog, Novolog, and Apidra are rapid-acting insulins.

47. B

Step 1: $\dfrac{25}{100} = \dfrac{1}{x}$

Step 2: $25x = 100$

Step 3: $x = 4$, therefore the ratio is 1:4.

48. A

A patient has gastroesophageal reflux disease if his/her profile lists the abbreviation "GERD."

49. D

Mupirocin is the generic name for Bactroban.

50. B

Transdermal patches should be applied to clean skin with minimal hair present. The skin should be free of powders, oils, and lotions. Transdermal patches should not be applied to broken skin.

51. A

USP <797> sets standards concerning the requirements for sterile preparation facilities.

52. B

Zestril is classified as an ACE inhibitor.

53. C

Unopened insulin should be stored in a refrigerator.

54. D

Fluticasone-salmeterol is the generic name for Advair.

55. C

Subcutaneous administration is the proper injection method for Lovenox.

56. A
Vitamin K plays a major role in blood clotting.

57. C
A reaction in which the actions of a drug are increased by the actions of another drug is a synergistic drug interaction.

58. C
A pharmacy registration with the DEA must be renewed every three years.

59. D
Step 1: $\dfrac{15\,g}{100\,g} = \dfrac{x\,g}{120\,g}$

Step 2: $100x = 1800$

Step 3: $x = 18\,g \times 1000 = 18{,}000$ mg

60. C
A suppository can be used vaginally or rectally.

61. B
A drug product that consists of a filthy, putrid, or decomposed substance would be in violation of the Food, Drug, and Cosmetic Act of 1938.

62. D
Gabapentin is the generic name for Neurontin.

63. C
Step 1: $25\% \times x$ mL $= 15\% \times 60$ mL
Step 2: $25x = 900$
Step 3: $x = 36$ mL

64. D
Patients on warfarin may have an increased bleeding risk if they are also taking aspirin, NSAIDs, or antiplatelets.

65. A
A laminar flow hood should be tested and certified every six months, whenever it is moved, or if the filter is damaged. Jewelry and artificial nails should not be worn in a laminar flow hood. Nothing should touch the HEPA filter.

66. D
Vitamins, herbs, and amino acids are considered dietary supplements by the FDA.

67. B
A "Store in Refrigerator" auxiliary label should be used with an Augmentin suspension.

68. A
Aleve, Motrin, and Advil are over-the-counter NSAIDs.

69. C
The abbreviation "gtt" represents "drop."

70. A
Sudafed is used for the treatment of nasal congestion.

71. A
No refills are permitted for a Schedule II controlled substance prescription.

72. C
A suspension is an example of a dispersion.

73. B
Deltasone is the brand name for prednisone.

74. B
Investigational New Drug Applications are reviewed by the FDA.

75. B
Among other duties, a pharmacy technician can update a patient profile, manage medication inventory, and bill a third-party provider.

76. D
An intradermal injection is administered into the top layer of skin.

77. B
Lotions contain the most amount of water of the dosage forms listed.

78. A
Norvasc, Cardizem, and Verelan are classified as calcium channel blockers.

79. A
Drug products that are considered to be therapeutically equivalent to other products will have a rating code that begins with the letter "A."

80. C
Ondansetron is used to treat nausea and vomiting.

81. B
Subcutaneous dosage forms should be injected under the skin.

82. A
Adderall, Vicodin, and OxyContin require a new prescription for each fill.

83. D
Air quality testing, product sterility testing, and the use of aseptic technique are required when compounding sterile products.

84. B
Furosemide is classified as a loop diuretic.

85. C
The sig "i cap po qod" translates to "Take one capsule by mouth every other day."

86. B
In a hospital, unit-dose carts consist of patient-specific medication.

87. B
An outpatient prescription label is required to include the number of refills authorized, the name of the drug manufacturer, and the name and address of the pharmacy.

88. A
Percocet is the brand name for oxycodone-acetaminophen.

89. A
Medications that are required to be frozen when stored should generally be kept within -25° and -10°C (-13 and 14°F).

90. C
Red yeast rice may help lower cholesterol levels.

91. C
A medication's expiration date is assigned by the drug manufacturer.

92. C
Hazardous waste is regulated by the Resource Conservation and Recovery Act.

93. A
Vicodin belongs to DEA Schedule II.

94. C
Glucophage is classified as a biguanide.

95. A
An "Avoid Prolonged Exposure to Sunlight" auxiliary label should be used with isotretinoin.

96. B
$$\frac{2 \text{ caps}}{\text{dose}} \times \frac{3 \text{ doses}}{\text{day}} \times 10 \text{ days} = 60 \text{ capsules}$$

97. B
Ditropan XL is the brand name for oxybutynin.

98. B
Flonase, Nasacort, and Zyrtec are available over the counter.

99. A
The beyond-use date for a high-risk compounded sterile product stored at room temperature cannot exceed 24 hours.

100. A
Heparin can be administered by the intravenous route.

ABOUT THE AUTHOR

Renee Bonsell is a staff pharmacist at an independent pharmacy in Columbus, Ohio. She earned her Doctor of Pharmacy degree from The Ohio State University in 2012, where she graduated summa cum laude. Renee is the author of the book "Pharmacy Technician Certification Exam Practice Question Workbook" and she currently holds a Certification in Delivering Medication Therapy Management Services, a Pharmacy-Based Immunization Certification, and a Basic Life Support Certification. In addition, Renee is a member of the Ohio Pharmacists Association and the American Pharmacists Association.

INDEX

CPSIA information can be obtained
at www.ICGtesting.com
Printed in the USA
FFHW01n0840170718
47463365-50704FF